Trauma and Disaster Responses and Management

Review of Psychiatry Series
John M. Oldham, M.D., M.S.
Michelle B. Riba, M.D., M.S.
Series Editors

Trauma and Disaster Responses and Management

EDITED BY

Robert J. Ursano, M.D.
Ann E. Norwood, M.D.

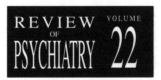

REVIEW OF PSYCHIATRY VOLUME 22

No. 1

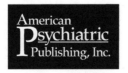

American Psychiatric Publishing, Inc.

Washington, DC
London, England

Copyright © 2003 American Psychiatric Publishing, Inc.
ALL RIGHTS RESERVED

Manufactured in the United States of America on acid-free paper
07 06 05 04 03   5 4 3 2 1
First Edition

Typeset in Adobe's Palatino

American Psychiatric Publishing, Inc.
1000 Wilson Boulevard
Arlington, VA 22209-3901
www.appi.org

The correct citation for this book is

Ursano R, Norwood AE (editors): *Trauma and Disaster Responses and Management* (Review of Psychiatry Series, Volume 22, Number 1; Oldham JM and Riba MB, series editors). Washington, DC, American Psychiatric Publishing, 2003

Library of Congress Cataloging-in-Publication Data
Trauma and disaster responses and management / edited by Robert J. Ursano, Ann E. Norwood.
    p. cm. — (Review of psychiatry ; . 22)
  Includes bibliographical references and index.
  ISBN 1-58562-115-3 (alk. paper)
    1. Psychic trauma—Treatment. 2. Post-traumatic stress disorder—Treatment. 3. Disasters—Psychological aspects. I. Ursano, Robert J., 1947– II. Norwood, Ann E., 1953–
III. Review of psychiatry series ; v. 22, no. 1.
RC552.P67T7355 2003
616.85′21—dc21

                                 2002043869

British Library Cataloguing in Publication Data
A CIP record is available from the British Library.

Contents

Chapter 5

Terrorism With Weapons of Mass Destruction: Chemical, Biological, Nuclear, Radiological, and Explosive Agents

Robert J. Ursano, M.D.
Ann E. Norwood, M.D.
Carol S. Fullerton, Ph.D.
Harry C. Holloway, M.D.
Molly Hall, M.D.

Contributors

Omer Bonne, M.D.
Senior Lecturer and Head of Outpatient Services, Department of Psychiatry, Hadassah University Hospital, Jerusalem, Israel; Research Fellow, Mood and Anxiety Disorders Program, National Institute of Mental Health, National Institutes of Health, Bethesda, Maryland

Dennis S. Charney, M.D.
Chief, Mood and Anxiety Disorders Program, National Institute of Mental Health, National Institutes of Health, Bethesda, Maryland

Spencer Eth, M.D.
Professor of Psychiatry, New York Medical College; Vice Chairman and Clinical Director, Department of Psychiatry, Saint Vincent's Hospital, New York, New York

Matthew J. Friedman, M.D., Ph.D.
Executive Director, National Center for PTSD, VA Regional Medical Center, White River Junction, Vermont

Carol S. Fullerton, Ph.D.
Research Associate Professor, Department of Psychiatry, F. Edward Hebert School of Medicine, Uniformed Services University of the Health Sciences, Bethesda, Maryland

Laura E. Gibson, Ph.D.
Clinical Assistant Professor, Department of Psychology, University of Vermont, Burlington, Vermont

Molly Hall, M.D.
Associate Professor, Department of Psychiatry, F. Edward Hebert School of Medicine, Uniformed Services University of the Health Sciences, Bethesda, Maryland

Harry C. Holloway, M.D.
Professor of Psychiatry and Neurosciences, Department of Psychiatry, F. Edward Hebert School of Medicine, Uniformed Services University of the Health Sciences, Bethesda, Maryland

Roy Lubit, M.D., Ph.D.
Assistant Professor, New York Medical College, Department of Psychiatry, Saint Vincent's Hospital, New York, New York

Alexander Neumeister, M.D.
Research Fellow, Mood and Anxiety Disorders Program, National Institute of Mental Health, National Institutes of Health, Bethesda, Maryland

Fran H. Norris, Ph.D.
Research Professor, Department of Psychiatry, Dartmouth Medical School; Disaster Research Coordinator, National Center for PTSD, White River Junction, Vermont

Carol S. North, M.D., M.P.E.
Professor, Department of Psychiatry, School of Medicine, Washington University, St. Louis, Missouri

Ann E. Norwood, M.D.
Associate Professor and Associate Chair, Department of Psychiatry, F. Edward Hebert School of Medicine, Uniformed Services University of the Health Sciences, Bethesda, Maryland

John M. Oldham, M.D., M.S.
Professor and Chair, Department of Psychiatry and Behavioral Sciences, Medical University of South Carolina, Charleston, South Carolina

Michelle B. Riba, M.D., M.S.
Clinical Professor and Associate Chair for Education and Academic Affairs, Department of Psychiatry, University of Michigan Medical School, Ann Arbor, Michigan

Elspeth Cameron Ritchie, M.D.
Director, Program Director, Mental Health Policy and Women's Issues, U.S. Department of Defense/Health Affairs, Falls Church, Virginia

Josef I. Ruzek, Ph.D.
Associate Director for Education, National Center for PTSD, Campbell, California

Robert J. Ursano, M.D.
Professor and Chairman, Department of Psychiatry, F. Edward Hebert School of Medicine, Uniformed Services University of the Health Sciences, Bethesda, Maryland

Patricia J. Watson, Ph.D.
Deputy for Education and Clinical Networking, National Center for PTSD, VA Regional Medical Center, White River Junction, Vermont

Introduction to the Review of Psychiatry Series

John M. Oldham, M.D., M.S.
Michelle B. Riba, M.D., M.S., Series Editors

2003 REVIEW OF PSYCHIATRY SERIES TITLES

- *Molecular Neurobiology for the Clinician*
  EDITED BY DENNIS S. CHARNEY, M.D.
- *Standardized Evaluation in Clinical Practice*
  EDITED BY MICHAEL B. FIRST, M.D.
- *Trauma and Disaster Responses and Management*
  EDITED BY ROBERT J. URSANO, M.D., AND
  ANN E. NORWOOD, M.D.
- *Geriatric Psychiatry*
  EDITED BY ALAN M. MELLOW, M.D., PH.D.

As our world becomes increasingly complex, we are learning more and living longer, yet we are presented with ever more complicated biological and psychosocial challenges. Packing into our heads all of the new things to know is a daunting task indeed. Keeping up with our children, all of whom learn to use computers and how to surf the Internet almost before they learn English, is even more challenging, but there is an excitement that accompanies these new languages that is sometimes almost breathtaking.

The explosion of knowledge in the field of molecular neurobiology charges ahead at breakneck speed, so that we have truly arrived at the technological doorway that is beginning to reveal the basic molecular and genetic fault lines of complex psychiatric diseases. In *Molecular Neurobiology for the Clinician*, edited by

Dr. Charney, Dr. McMahon (Chapter 2) outlines a number of genetic discoveries that have the potential to affect our clinical practice in important ways, such as validating diagnostic systems and disease entities, improving treatment planning, and developing novel therapies and preventive interventions. Examples of these principles are illustrated in this book as they apply to addictive disorders (Chapter 4, by Dr. Nestler), schizophrenia (Chapter 3, by Dr. Gilbert and colleagues), psychiatric disorders of childhood and adolescence (Chapter 1, by Drs. Veenstra-VanderWeele and Cook), and mood and anxiety disorders (Chapter 5, by Dr. Gould and colleagues).

Increased precision and standardization characterizes not only the microworld of research but also the macroworld of clinical practice. Current recommendations regarding standardized assessment in clinical practice are reviewed in *Standardized Evaluation in Clinical Practice,* edited by Dr. First, recognizing that we must be prepared to reshape our diagnostic ideas based on new evidence from molecular genetics and neurobiology, as well as from the findings of clinical research itself. In Chapter 1, Dr. Basco outlines a number of problems inherent in routine clinical diagnostic practice, including inaccurate or incomplete diagnoses, omission of comorbidities, and various sources of bias, and an argument is made to train clinicians in the use of a standardized diagnostic method, such as the *Structured Clinical Interview for DSM* (SCID). Similar problems are reviewed by Dr. Lucas (Chapter 3) in work with child and adolescent patients, and a self-report diagnostic assessment technique, the Computerized Diagnostic Interview Schedule for Children (CDISC), is described. The CDISC is reported to have the advantages of enhancing patients' abilities to discuss their concerns and enhanced caretaker satisfaction with the intake interview.

Similarly, Dr. Zimmerman (Chapter 2) underscores the importance of developing a standardized clinical measure with good psychometric properties that could be incorporated into routine clinical practice, presenting data suggesting the value of one such system, the Rhode Island Method to Improve Diagnostic Assessment and Services (MIDAS) project. Dr. Oquendo and colleagues (Chapter 4), in turn, review the critical issue of the use of standardized scales to enhance detection of suicidal behavior and risk of suicide in individual patients. The challenge to establish the cost-effectiveness of standardized assessment methodology in clinical practice is illustrated by the efforts in the U.S. Department of Veterans Affairs system, described by Dr. Van Stone and colleagues (Chapter 5), to train clinicians in the use of the Global Assessment of Functioning (GAF) scale, and to incorporate it into the electronic medical record.

In *Trauma and Disaster Responses and Management*, edited by Drs. Ursano and Norwood, a compelling case is made by Dr. Bonne and colleagues (Chapter 1) of the fundamental interconnectedness between lifelong biological processes in humans and animals, and the environment. The relevance of studies using animal models to our understanding of posttraumatic stress disorder and other stress syndromes has become increasingly important, elucidating the functional neuroanatomy and neuroendocrinology of stress responses. This growing research database proves compelling when contemplating the human impact of major disasters such as the Oklahoma City bombing, described by Dr. North (Chapter 2), the effect of the World Trade Center tragedy and other disasters on developing children, described by Drs. Lubit and Eth (Chapter 3), and the potential and actual impact of bioterrorism on individuals and large populations, reviewed by Dr. Ursano and colleagues (Chapter 5). The need for early intervention, articulated by Dr. Watson and colleagues (Chapter 4), becomes increasingly clear as we learn more, which we must, about trauma and its effects.

As we learn more about many things, we make progress, but always with a cost. We are getting better at fighting illness and preserving health, hence we live longer. With longer life, however, comes new challenges, such as preserving the quality of life during these extended years. *Geriatric Psychiatry*, edited by Dr. Mellow, focuses on the growing field of geriatric psychiatry, from the points of view of depression (Chapter 1, by Dr. Mellow), dementia (Chapter 2, by Dr. Weiner), psychoses (Chapter 3, by Drs. Grossberg and Desai), late-life addictions (Chapter 4, by Drs. Blow and Oslin), and public policy (Chapter 5, by Dr. Colenda and colleagues). It is clear that we are making progress in diagnosis and treatment of all of these conditions that accompany our increased longevity; it is also clear that in the future we will increasingly emphasize prevention of illness and health-promoting habits and behaviors. Because understanding motivated behavior is a mainstay of what psychiatry is all about and we still have not unraveled all of the reasons why humans do things that are bad for them, business will be brisk.

Continuing our tradition of presenting a selection of topics in each year's Review of Psychiatry Series that includes new research findings and new developments in clinical care, we look forward to Volume 23 in the Review of Psychiatry Series, which will feature brain stimulation in psychiatric treatment (edited by Sarah H. Lisanby, M.D.), developmental psychobiology (edited by B.J. Casey, Ph.D.), medical laboratory and neuropsychiatric testing (edited by Stuart C. Yudofsky, M.D., and H. Florence Kim, M.D.), and cognitive-behavioral therapy (edited by Jesse H. Wright III, M.D., Ph.D.).

Preface

Robert J. Ursano, M.D.
Ann E. Norwood, M.D.

In this book in the Review of Psychiatry series, the impact of trauma is examined from the cellular to the community level. Distress after traumatic events such as September 11 is universal. For most people, transient sleep disturbance, increased anxiety, preoccupation with the event, traumatic reminders, emotional numbness, and social withdrawal will dissipate over time. For others, however, symptoms do not resolve, and a range of psychiatric disorders ensue.

In their chapter, Drs. Bonne, Neumeister, and Charney discuss the neurobiological and neuroanatomical responses to severe traumatic events and the process by which an initially adaptive response becomes maladaptive, producing long-term adverse consequences. The authors approach the neural mechanisms of posttraumatic stress disorder (PTSD) by presenting data touching on the major symptom clusters of reexperiencing, avoidance, and increased arousal.

Dr. Carol North provides a review of the psychiatric epidemiology of disaster. In this comprehensive chapter, Dr. North examines individual and community responses to disasters as an empirical basis for the development of interventions. She notes the high frequency of comorbid disorders that can affect the course of recovery from PTSD and that may influence the choice of treatments for PTSD. Her examination of vulnerabilities for psychiatric disorders can help guide the psychiatrist in identifying and following up high-risk groups.

Drs. Roy Lubit and Spencer Eth review the impact of traumatic stressors on children. They debunk the myth that children are more resilient than adults in the wake of catastrophe. For children, trauma can disrupt normal development and can create a series of secondary adversities such as poor school performance. Children's dependency on adults makes them vulnerable to the ways in which parents and teachers cope with the tragedy. The authors present a thorough review of pertinent literature on children's responses to trauma gleaned across national and international events. They illustrate many of their points with observations and findings from the September 11, 2001, attack on the World Trade Center. Finally, they present a compelling case for the need to improve the delivery of mental health services to traumatized children.

Drs. Watson, Friedman, Gibson, Ruzek, Norris, and Ritchie present material from an international consensus conference on psychological interventions following mass violence. The authors begin by reviewing data on the psychological impact of disasters, focusing on risk and protective factors. They then provide a detailed review of scientific data on acute interventions for trauma, examining psychological debriefing, the treatment of traumatic grief, pharmacotherapy, cognitive-behavioral therapy, and interventions for children.

Finally, the special dilemmas posed by traumatic stress caused by chemical, biological, nuclear, radiological, and high-yield explosive (CBNRE) agents are reviewed by Drs. Ursano, Norwood, Fullerton, Holloway, and Hall. The events of September 11 and the subsequent anthrax attacks brought the psychological and behavioral responses to terrorism into sharp relief. This chapter discusses attributes of CBNRE agents that make them especially effective as instruments of terror against individuals and communities. The Tokyo sarin attack, the SCUD missile attacks against Israel during the Persian Gulf War, and a radiation accident in Goiania, Brazil, are used as case examples. Recommendations are made on ways in which nations can enhance preparedness for the psychological and behavioral toll of these novel weapons.

These authors summarize current understanding of the complex psychological, behavioral, and social responses to disaster. Although we have learned much from past experience, these authors remind us of the need for a continued focus on service delivery and on basic science and intervention outcomes research.

Chapter 1

Neurobiological Mechanisms of Psychological Trauma

Omer Bonne, M.D.
Alexander Neumeister, M.D.
Dennis S. Charney, M.D.

Phenomenology and Classification

In DSM-IV-TR (American Psychiatric Association 2000), a traumatic event is defined as one that involves a threat of death or physical integrity to self or others and results in a subjective response of fear, helplessness, or horror. Epidemiological research has revealed that up to 90% of citizens in the United States are exposed to at least one traumatic event (as defined in DSM-IV-TR) in the course of their lives (Breslau and Kessler 2001), and many of these individuals are exposed to more than one traumatic event.

This chapter focuses on the biology of the response to trauma. Data gathered from clinical and preclinical research demonstrate a uniquely homogeneous response to acute exposure to trauma in both biology and phenomenology. Thus, the initial physiological response to threat should be considered a normal adaptive survival mechanism. However, short- and long-term sequelae of exposure to trauma vary greatly, ranging from complete recovery to severe and debilitating posttraumatic stress disorder (PTSD). In this chapter we first describe the phenomenology of the acute response to severe trauma and the clinical picture of PTSD. We then examine the way acute and chronic stress reactions are addressed by the current categorical diagnostic system. The focus of this chapter, however, is on the neurobiology and neuroanatomy of the response to severe traumatic events, their long-term consequences, and the process whereby an initially adaptive response becomes maladaptive and harmful.

Acute Stress Response, Acute Stress Disorder, Acute and Chronic PTSD

A typical pattern of mental, emotional, and physical response is observed in the majority of people after exposure to severe trauma. This response consists of increased anxiety and arousal; sleep difficulties; emotional numbness and withdrawal; and preoccupation with and reexperiencing of the outstanding event. In most people exposed to trauma, the severity of response will diminish, beginning within days or weeks of exposure. This may explain why, by definition, the diagnosis of PTSD can be conferred no earlier than a month after exposure to the traumatic event. Still, signs of psychopathology can already be observed well before the end of the first month after trauma. Severely traumatized survivors describe a sense of profound transformation: their mood is dysphoric and irritable, they have lost their sense of safety, and they scan the outside world for potential threats. Sleep is of poor quality and is disturbed by nightmares. Harmony with others and within oneself seems to have been lost. Relationships are troubled by outbursts of anger, a tendency to isolate oneself, and inability to share inner experiences. Such symptoms often herald the onset of psychopathology. Early responses effectively communicate a need for help. However, premature psychological intervention may be harmful, possibly because it can interfere with drawing on personal support systems and normal recovery. Disentangling adaptive components from harmful components of the early stress response is therefore a major challenge.

The somewhat controversial diagnosis of acute stress disorder (ASD), introduced in DSM-IV (American Psychiatric Association 1994), addresses psychopathology within 2 days and 1 month of exposure to trauma. This diagnosis is phenomenologically similar to that of PTSD, consisting of its three symptom clusters, with the addition of a disparate symptom cluster consisting of five dissociative phenomena. The presence of three such symptoms is mandatory for the diagnosis of ASD, making dissociation a major and core symptom requirement in this new entity, in contrast to PTSD. The requirement for dissociative symptoms seemed too restrictive to some authors, who showed that categorizing early pathological stress response according to symptoms other than dissociation is no less effective in predicting PTSD (Brewin et al. 1999). Several additional factors increase the likelihood of developing ASD and PTSD, such as increased severity and duration of trauma exposure, female gender, a subjective feeling that life is threatened, overidentifying with victims, and peritraumatic depressive symptoms. Physiological predictors of PTSD have also been proposed (and confirmed), such as having an elevated heart rate at the emergency room.

The severity of the stress response reflects the intensity and configuration of the stressor. Events associated with torture or prolonged victimization are associated with the highest estimates for chronic PTSD. Still, even among those who are exposed to severe and prolonged trauma, a substantial number will not develop PTSD. Thus, PTSD can be considered a possible, but not an inevitable, outcome of trauma exposure. ASD is diagnosed in 15%–20% of survivors of civilian trauma (Brewin et al. 1999). A majority (up to 80%) of persons with a diagnosis of ASD still experience PTSD at 6 months, and most of these will also harbor the disorder 2 years after exposure. Yet many survivors who do not meet diagnostic criteria for ASD will develop PTSD.

After the 1-month time limit for ASD, symptomatic patients are given a diagnosis of acute PTSD until 3 months after the trauma. Any trauma-related psychopathology after this period meeting criteria for PTSD is diagnosed as chronic PTSD. In a minority of subjects, symptoms of PTSD will only appear long after exposure to trauma. When this time lag is at least 6 months, a diagnosis of PTSD with a delayed onset is applied.

Resilience

The risk of incurring PTSD increases with the severity of trauma. With regard to PTSD, resilience is defined as the capacity to withstand extreme stress or trauma without developing pathological symptoms. Current research has involved extensive study of PTSD and attempts to identify vulnerability and risk factors, but no investigations of resilience have been undertaken. Methodologically sound research of resilience is complex and would ideally entail a prospective investigation of individuals before exposure to trauma. Given the obvious difficulties in carrying out such studies, recent research has included investigations of persons in high-risk, trauma-exposed professions, such as army personnel (particularly members of elite units), firefighters, police officers, and emergency medicine personnel. Researchers sought associations between mental status or performance during and after exposure to severe stress and psychosocial or biological measures. Research is seminal, and results have varied widely. Notably, in a series of studies Morgan et al. (2001) suggested that levels of neuropeptide Y are positively associated with performance and emotional state during and soon after exposure to uncontrollable stress.

Neural Mechanism and Functional Neuroanatomy of PTSD

PTSD is a devastating and chronic disorder and is often resistant to treatment. In DSM-IV-TR, PTSD symptoms are grouped into three broad categories (American Psychiatric Association 2000): 1) reexperiencing (i.e., persistent involuntary thoughts and dreams of the traumatic event, accompanied by psychological distress); 2) avoidance of stimuli associated with the trauma, numbing, and interpersonal constriction; and 3) increased arousal (sleep difficulties, irritability, hypervigilance and exaggerated startle reactivity, and difficulty concentrating). For clarity, in this discussion neural mechanisms of PTSD are linked to symptom clusters. This should not be understood to imply that symptom clusters are separate or independent.

Reexperiencing

Conditioning

In patients with PTSD, the traumatic event persistently intrudes into awareness. Vivid memories of the trauma and correspond-

---

ing stressful emotional responses are triggered by external or internal, often unremarkable, stimuli. Reexperiencing may involve thoughts, perceptions, images, and dreams. In severe cases, patients may act or feel as if they are actually reliving the traumatic experience, at times losing orientation to time and place.

Conditioned fear responses, studied mostly (but not exclusively) in rodents, have been suggested as a model for the reexperiencing phenomena in PTSD (LeDoux 2000; Maren 2001). Studies have shown that fear conditioning is very rapidly acquired (Maren 2001), with often a single exposure to a pairing of an unconditioned stimulus (US) and a conditioned stimulus (CS) sufficing to induce a conditioned response (CR) to a CS (LeDoux 2000). Animal studies have additionally shown that fear conditioning may be very persistent, with the CS-CR coupling remaining potentially active indefinitely (LeDoux 2000; Maren 2001). During fear conditioning, the animal learns that the CS (to be termed CS+) predicts the US. When a different neutral CS is consistently not followed by a US (termed CS–), it would be understood as a safety signal. Alternation between CS+ and CS– is termed differential fear conditioning. *Extinction* refers to the process whereby conditioned fear responses (CRs) are reduced when the CS is no longer reinforced by the aversive US. In contrast with earlier theories, the reduction of fear that follows extinction does not result from forgetting or memory erasure. Rather, it involves the formation of new associations that compete with the prior fear-conditioned associations (Bouton 1988). The conditioned association is not erased, and it may be reactivated under particular circumstances after extinction. Examples of such reactivated conditioning are the renewal of fear conditioning if a CS is presented in a context different from the one in which extinction was performed or the reinstatement of fear conditioning on pairing of the CS with even a mild US (Bouton 1988).

As described, most people who are exposed to a traumatic event exhibit temporary PTSD-like distress but do not develop PTSD (Breslau and Kessler 2001). Bearing in mind the conditioning model, we hypothesize that 1) fear conditioning occurs in the majority of subjects exposed to an intense traumatic event; 2) the normal healthy response after surviving a traumatic experience is an extinction (-like) process, beginning soon after the trauma, resulting in a gradual uncoupling of the CS-CR; and 3) PTSD is mainly a result of impaired extinction.

In animals, extinction of fear conditioning is a much more time-consuming process than acquisition of fear conditioning (LeDoux 2000). Although this is not necessarily true for humans, this time frame is compatible with normal acute stress reaction phenomenology, with gradual decline in distress beginning within the first days and continuing for weeks and sometimes months after trauma. The concept of extinction as a competitive learning process rather than memory erasure is also compatible with PTSD phenomenology: it may explain why the foremost vulnerability factor for acquisition of PTSD is history of trauma and abuse. It may also help to explain the occurrence of delayed PTSD. In addition, even apparently asymptomatic patients with (past) PTSD respond with an intense emotional reaction when faced with circumstances even remotely similar to their index trauma.

Patients with PTSD reexperience in response to a variety of trauma-related, non-trauma-related, and poorly defined internal stimuli. This may be understood as a failure in differential conditioning and is termed *generalization*. As PTSD progresses to chronicity, patients experience an elevated baseline (anticipatory) level of anxiety. This occurs when patients with PTSD have learned that aversive emotional experiences are both inevitable and unpredictable.

Memory

A large body of evidence suggests that arousing, fearful, or emotionally exciting events are remembered better and for longer periods of time than emotionally neutral events (McGaugh 2000). It has been hypothesized that the release of cortisol, epinephrine, and norepinephrine after trauma exposure causes an overconsolidation of memory for the stressful event (Roozendaal 2000). Animal data have shown that administration of cortisol, epinephrine, and norepinephrine enhances both consolidation of memory and memory retrieval (for reviews, see McGaugh and Roozendaal 2002; Southwick et al. 1999a).

Because traumatic events indeed stimulate release of cortisol and catecholamine, the result could be a deeply engraved traumatic memory that is clinically expressed in the form of intrusive recollections, flashbacks, and repetitive nightmares, perhaps facilitating conditioned emotional responses. A positive feedback loop would be formed, because every time the traumatic memory is vividly reexperienced, cortisol, epinephrine, and norepinephrine are released, further strengthening the memory trace and increasing the likelihood of subsequent intrusive recollections (McGaugh 2000).

Neurocircuitry of Reexperiencing

Integration of CSs and USs and the resultant fear conditioning and response are mediated by the amygdala and its projections (LeDoux 2000). Cue CSs are transmitted by external and visceral sensory pathways to the thalamus. Afferents then reach the basolateral amygdala via two parallel neural circuits: a rapid subcortical path (the short loop) directly from the dorsal (sensory) thalamus, and a slower regulatory cortical pathway (the long loop) encompassing the primary somatosensory cortices, the insula, and the anterior cingulate and prefrontal cortices (LeDoux 2000). Context CSs are projected to the lateral amygdala from the hippocampus (Phillips and LeDoux 1992) and perhaps also from the bed nucleus of the stria terminalis (BNST) (M. Davis et al. 1997). Human subjects with lesions of the amygdala and adjacent regions show impaired fear conditioning. Pathways conveying the US have not been studied as much but are believed to reach the basolateral and central nucleus of the amygdala from the thalamus, parabrachial area, spinal cord, and somatosensory cortical regions (LeDoux 2000).

Less is currently known about neuroanatomy and mechanisms of extinction. Opinions differ regarding the roles of the medial prefrontal cortex (LeDoux 2000) and the amygdala (M. Davis et al. 1997) in this process. Activity of the right prefrontal cortex was shown to be inversely correlated with activity of the amygdala, suggesting an inhibitory modulatory influence.

Human functional magnetic resonance imaging (fMRI) studies in healthy subjects show fear conditioning–related activation in the amygdala, anterior cingulate cortex, and precentral regions (Buchel et al. 1998; LaBar et al. 1998). Positron emission tomographic studies of aversive conditioning do not depict involvement of the amygdala in fear conditioning but rather describe activation of diverse cortical regions, such as anterior cingulate cortex precentral and premotor regions, and orbitofrontal, prefrontal, and temporal cortices.

The amygdala is also implicated in memory processing of particularly emotionally arousing events (McGaugh 2000). Lesions of the amygdala block the enhancing effects of emotional arousal on memory consolidation as well as the memory-modulatory effects of systemic administration of catecholamines and cortisol (Roozendaal 2000). These effects are mediated by the basolateral nucleus of the amygdala and the BNST.

Functional imaging studies in PTSD show right amygdala activation when patients and control subjects were exposed to traumatic imagery and pictures, whereas the left amygdala was activated in response to sounds. Such studies also show decreased perfusion in the anterior cingulate cortex in patients with PTSD after traumatic memory provocation. Recent fMRI studies similarly show reduced perfusion in the anterior cingulate cortex in patients with PTSD compared with control subjects after emotional provocation (for review, see Pitman et al. 2001).

Avoidance, Numbing, and Interpersonal Constriction

The second major cluster of symptoms in PTSD is composed of avoidance of stimuli associated with the trauma and emotional numbing, leading to social withdrawal.

Fear response is at once conditioned to both an explicit cue (cue conditioning) and the environment where the cue was delivered (contextual conditioning) (Phillips and LeDoux 1992). Whereas cue conditioning results in the episodic localized fear response, contextual fear conditioning is said to capture characteristics of sustained anxiety as well. Avoidance can be understood as a consequence of contextual conditioning: patients with PTSD learn that they have a high risk of a fear response at certain circumstances and avoid these conditions as much as possible (similar to the agoraphobic behavior of many patients with panic disorder), leading to a restricted behavioral pattern. Avoidance then deteriorates due to the generalization of fear response (as described under Conditioning) until social withdrawal is almost complete.

The interpersonal deficits within this cluster are phenomenologically similar to depressive symptoms and may partly represent the high comorbidity between PTSD and depression (Breslau and Kessler 2001). *Learned helplessness* is a description of animal behavior after exposure to inescapable stress (Maier 2001). Inescapable stress is used to generate animal models for anxiety-depression spectrum disorders, including PTSD. The behavioral syndrome after inescapable stress includes social withdrawal, reduced food and liquid intake, and reduced aggressiveness. Inescapable stress enhances fear conditioning (Maier 2001) and results in poor escape learning on exposure to subsequent stress. Although this behavioral pattern typically lasts for a few days, exposing rats to the environment in which the inescapable stress had occurred prolongs the behavioral syndrome indefinitely.

Neurocircuitry of Avoidance, Numbing, and Interpersonal Constriction

Whereas cued fear is predominantly modulated by the amygdala, the amygdala, hippocampus, and BNST are all involved in contextual fear conditioning (Phillips and LeDoux 1992; Walker and Davis 1997). The BNST, a small nucleus situated between several other nuclei that make up the ventral striatum, has been specifically implicated in more sustained states of anxiety (Walker and Davis 1997). It is an important relay station that links the amygdala and hippocampus with regions of the paraventricular nucleus (PVN) of the hypothalamus and the brain stem (M. Davis et al. 1997), suggesting a central role for this structure in anxiety regulation.

The neural circuitry of learned helplessness is still unclear. Levels of 5-hydroxytryptamine (5-HT) (serotonin) after inescapable stress are increased in the basolateral nucleus of the amygdala (Amat et al. 1998). A preliminary neuronal network of learned helplessness, been proposed (Petty et al. 1997) that includes brain stem nuclei (locus coeruleus [LC], dorsal raphe, ventral tegmental nucleus), limbic system (entorhinal cortex, hippocampus, septum, hypothalamus), and medial prefrontal cortex (mPFC).

Increased Arousal

The hyperarousal symptom cluster comprises symptoms suggestive of persistent baseline anxiety as well as autonomic and motor hyperresponsivity to sudden neutral stimuli. PTSD patients experience sleep difficulties, difficulty concentrating, irritability, and hypervigilance. They also exhibit elevated baseline heart rate, increased skin conductance and slower skin conductance response habituation, exaggerated startle reactivity, and reduction of the P200 response to loud sounds (Orr and Roth 2000). Rauch et al. (2000) reported exaggerated amygdala responses to mask-fearful versus mask-happy faces in patients with PTSD compared with those of combat-exposed veterans without PTSD. This is suggestive of a discrete amygdala abnormality in PTSD.

The concept of sensitization has been suggested as a model for the hyperarousal symptoms in PTSD. Sensitization is defined as an elementary form of nonassociative learning in which an animal learns to strengthen its defensive reflexes and to respond vigorously to a variety of previously neutral or indifferent stimuli after it has been exposed to a potentially threatening or noxious stimulus (Kandel and Schwartz 1982). Sensitization may be relevant to the irritability, hypervigilance, and exaggerated startle reactivity of PTSD. Sensitization may also contribute to the vulnerability for PTSD in individuals with childhood trauma exposure (Heim and Nemeroff 2001).

Another phenomenon related to the hyperarousal cluster is the delay in (or absence of) habituation often reported in PTSD. In healthy individuals, repeated presentation of stimuli leads to a progressive reduction of initially increased regional cerebral blood flow in brain areas involved in the processing of these stimuli (e.g., amygdala and hippocampus) (Breiter and Rauch 1996; Buchel et al. 1998). Habituation of the amygdala was not reported for patients with PTSD who were exposed to repeated exposure (Rauch et al. 2000). Patients with PTSD also show a delay in habituation of skin conductance responses to acoustic startle (Orr and Roth 2000).

Neurocircuitry of Increased Arousal

The state of increased arousal can be regarded as an extended nonconditioned fear response. This response originates in the amygdala and the BNST. Efferent projections from the amygdala reach the LC, hypothalamus, dorsal motor nerve root of the vagus nerve and nucleus ambiguus, parabrachial nucleus, periaqueductal gray matter, hippocampus, striatum, and brain stem nuclei (M. Davis et al. 1997; LeDoux 2000). Projections from the BNST to autonomic regulatory brain stem areas include the LC, nucleus tractus solitarius, caudal ventrolateral medulla, and dorsal nucleus of the vagus, supporting a role for the BNST in the control of arousal and autonomic responses. Lesioning the BNST with N-methyl-D-aspartate (NMDA) and administering corticotropin-releasing hormone (CRH) antagonist to the BNST blocked CRH-enhanced (but not fear-potentiated) startle. In animals with amygdala lesions, the opposite pattern was observed (Lee and Davis 1997). In light of the high cerebrospinal fluid levels of CRH observed in PTSD, this finding suggests a major role for the BNST in PTSD.

The anterior cingulate cortex has extensive connections with brain regions involved in arousal and regulation of the autonomic nervous system. The exact nature of this association has not been fully elucidated. Malfunction of the anterior cingulate cortex, as postulated before, may be involved in the attenuated habituation and psychophysiological arousal (Orr and Roth. 2000) seen in PTSD. The neural circuitry mediating sensitization is believed to include the dopaminergic neuronal system in the nucleus accumbens, striatum, mPFC, hypothalamus, and amygdala; noradrenergic neurotransmission in the LC, hypothalamus, amygdala, and hippocampus; and NMDA receptor modulation in the amygdala and prefrontal cortex (Charney et al. 1993).

Animal studies have been conducted in which preshocked rats were exposed to moderate novel stress. Compared with never-shocked control rats, the preshocked rats had significantly higher numbers of neurons containing early gene activation markers in many brain areas: nucleus accumbens, BNST, basolateral amygdala, hippocampus, PVN of the hypothalamus, LC, and others (Bruijnzeel et al. 1999). In similarly designed studies, postsensitization exposure to moderate stress induced a significant increase in CRH immunoreactivity in the PVN of the hypothalamus, the median eminence, and the central amygdala (Bruijnzeel et al. 2001). Exposure to inescapable stress (described under Avoidance, Numbing, and Interpersonal Constriction) also results in a long-lasting sensitization, as observed by an increased startle response to auditory tones (Servatius et al. 1994).

Stress and the Hippocampus

The hippocampal formation is highly vulnerable to insults such as stroke, seizures, head trauma, and psychological stress. In addition, the volume of the hippocampus is largely determined by heredity (Lyons et al. 2001). Neurotoxic damage to the hippocampus and suppression of ongoing neurogenesis are direct consequences of glucocorticoid administration (reviewed in McEwen 2000) and are augmented by the presence of glutamate and glutamate analogs such as NMDA. Psychosocial stress also induces hippocampal neurotoxicity and volume loss. Glucocorticoid increase in response to environmental stressors is well documented. Animal studies have likewise shown immediate glutamate efflux in prefrontal cortex and hippocampus after induction of acute stress (Bagley and Moghaddam 1997). Hippocampal atrophy is blocked by inhibiting the formation of adrenal steroids and by blocking the actions of excitatory amino acids using phenytoin or NMDA receptor inhibitors (McEwen 2000). Recent research has also demonstrated that stress-induced changes in cerebral metabolites, hippocampal volume, and cell proliferation are prevented by treatment with the antidepressant tianeptine (Czeh et al. 2001).

Stress-induced hippocampal volume reduction in animals is apparently the measurable outcome of several pathological processes (e.g., reduction of dendrite length in pyramidal and granule neurons, suppression of dentate granular cell neurogenesis, and neuronal and glial neurotoxic cell loss) (McEwen 2000). Animal studies indicate that most such hippocampal damage is reversible. Evidently, the issue of reversibility has not been adequately examined in human subjects. However, Starkman et al. (1999) reported an increase in hippocampal volume after correction of the hypercortisolism of Cushing's syndrome. In addition to Cushing's syndrome (and PTSD), reduced hippocampal volume has been reported in humans with major depression, normal aging, and dementia, suggesting that this phenomenon may not be related to any specific mental disorder but rather to prolonged insult.

Recent work has assigned an explicit role for the dorsal hippocampus in mediating PTSD-associated behaviors such as spatial learning, fear conditioning, and appetitive instrumental conditioning. Downregulation of brain-derived neurotrophic factor (BDNF) mRNA in the dentate gyrus of the hippocampus was reported in animals exposed to an unconditioned stressor and lately also in animals that were reexposed to traumatic cues (Rasmusson et al. 2002). BDNF is a member of the neurotrophin family of peptides and has been shown to support neuronal growth, differentiation, and survival in the developing and the adult hippocampus. Decreased expression of BDNF is hypothesized to play a role in the atrophy of hippocampal neurons in experimental animals in response to stress. Reexposure to trauma-related cues may thus disrupt the formation of associations such as those required by extinction and may thereby undermine the efficacy of exposure therapy in some individuals with PTSD.

Neuroimaging Studies in PTSD

Amygdala activation was observed in patients with PTSD after traumatic provocation. However, this activation was often similar in subjects with PTSD and in control subjects without PTSD who had experienced trauma. The absence of group difference may reflect limitations in statistical sensitivity or in the temporal resolution of nuclear imaging. Thus, a preliminary fMRI study found higher hemodynamic changes in the amygdala in subjects with PTSD relative to matched trauma-exposed control subjects without PTSD during exposure to mask-fearful faces (for review, see Pitman et al. 2001). Other limbic and paralimbic cortical structures have also been implicated in functional imaging of PTSD. In both subjects with PTSD and matched trauma-exposed control subjects without PTSD, increases in cerebral blood flow (CBF) were found in the posterior orbital cortex, anterior insula, and temporopolar cortex during exposure to trauma-related stimuli. In contrast, the pattern of changes elicited in the mPFC by traumatic stimuli may differ between subjects with PTSD and control subjects. Thus, regional CBF decreased in the left but increased in the right pregenual anterior cingulate cortex in PTSD, suggesting that the role of the mPFC in emotional behavior is lateralized. However, CBF in the right pregenual anterior cingulate cortex increased significantly more in non-PTSD, trauma-matched control subjects than in PTSD subjects. Moreover, in the infralimbic cortex, CBF decreased in combat-related PTSD subjects but increased in combat-matched, non-PTSD control subjects during exposure to combat-related visual and auditory stimuli (Pitman et al. 2001). Two recent fMRI studies show reduced perfusion in the anterior cingulate cortex in PTSD subjects compared with that in trauma-exposed control subjects after activation by emotional Stroop task (Shin et al. 2001) and traumatic recall (Lanius et al. 2001). The observation that PTSD subjects do not activate the anterior cingulate cortex supports the hypothesis that neural processes mediating extinction may be impaired in PTSD.

Structural imaging investigation of hippocampal volume in PTSD was largely stimulated by preclinical studies reporting hippocampal neuronal loss and dendritic atrophy following exposure to hydrocortisone or psychosocial stress in rats, as described under Increased Arousal. MRI studies of PTSD have identified subtle reductions in the volume of the hippocampus in PTSD samples relative to healthy or traumatized non-PTSD control samples (for review, see Villarreal and King 2001; Villarreal et al. 2002). Although limitations existed in these studies in the matching of alcohol use between PTSD and control samples, the reductions in hippocampal volume did not correlate with the extent of alcohol exposure. Volume reductions were associated with short-term memory deficits (Villarreal and King 2001). In contrast, a recent MRI study (Schuff et al. 2001) found no difference in hippocampal volume between patients and control subjects. Moreover, prospective longitudinal studies of acutely traumatized adult survivors (Bonne et al. 2001) and children (De Bellis et al. 2001) found no difference in hippocampal volume between healthy trauma survivors and PTSD patients. The reason for this difference between studies is unclear.

Neuroendocrinology and Neurochemistry of Stress and PTSD

Activation of the neuroanatomical circuits described is dependent on a variety of neuroendocrine systems for both neurotransmission and modulation. Neurochemicals include the peptidergic neurotransmitters CRH and neuropeptide Y; opiates; the monoaminergic transmitters norepinephrine, serotonin, and dopamine; and the amino acid transmitters γ-aminobutyric acid (GABA) and arginine vasopressin (AVP). The neurotransmitter systems that have been best studied in association with responses to stress or threat involve the hypothalamic-pituitary-adrenal (HPA) axis and the central noradrenergic system. These systems prepare the organism to respond to threat or stress by increasing vigilance, modulating memory, mobilizing energy stores, increasing cardiovascular function, and planning and preparing motor responses. However, these normally adaptive responses can become maladaptive if their regulation is impaired. The preclinical and clinical literature regarding these neurochemical concomitants of stress and fear and their potential relevance to the pathophysiology PTSD are reviewed in the following section.

HPA Axis and CRH: Activity and Regulation

Corticosteroid hormones (mainly cortisol in humans and corticosterone in rodents) are lipophilic molecules that are secreted in response to stress by the adrenal gland and follow a circadian pattern. HPA axis function is regulated via feedback of glucocorticoids at the level of the pituitary, hypothalamus, and suprahypothalamic limbic compartments such as the hippocampus, mPFC, and amygdala. The feedback inhibition of CRH function by glucocorticoids occurs at the level of the PVN of the hypothalamus (where systemically administered glucocorticoids reduce CRH expression) and the anterior pituitary (where glucocorticoids decrease CRH receptor expression). In contrast, glucocorticoids and stress apparently provide positive feedback on extrahypothalamic CRH function in the amygdala or the BNST that may contribute to the production of anxiety symptoms (Schulkin et al. 1998). Glucocorticoid signals are transduced via heterogeneous corticosteroid nuclear receptors known as type 1 or mineralocorticoid receptors and type 2 or glucocorticoid receptors.

Mineralocorticoid receptors have a higher affinity but a lower capacity for cortisol, are thought to be mostly occupied by cortisol at all times, and provide a basal glucocorticoid tone. Glucocorticoid receptors have a lower affinity and greater capacity for cortisol and are assumed to play a leading part in stress response once cortisol levels increase. Glucocorticoid receptors have particularly high densities in areas related to stress responses such as the hypothalamus, the serotoninergic and noradrenergic cell bodies, and the hippocampus. Mineralocorticoid expression is mainly in limbic brain regions such as the hippocampus, septum, and amygdala in rodents.

Exposure to stress of various types results in a release of CRH, adrenocorticotropic hormone (ACTH), and cortisol. This HPA-axis activation during episodes of acute stress can result in transient elevation of the plasma concentration of cortisol and partial resistance to feedback inhibition of cortisol release that persists during and shortly after the duration of the stressful stimulus. This phenomenon may produce a rapid downregulation of glucocorticoid receptors, resulting in increased corticosterone secretion and feedback resistance. After termination of the stress, glucocorticoid receptor density increases and feedback sensitivity normalizes (Korte 2001). Functional differences between CRH receptor subtypes may also contribute to the modulation of stress response. CRH type 1 and CRH type 2 receptors appear to play reciprocal roles in mediating stress responsiveness and behavior. Regional differences in the anatomical distribution of CRH type 1 and CRH type 2 receptors are likely to play a role in balancing facilitatory versus modulatory effects of CRH receptor stimulation on stress responses (for review, see Reul and Holsboer 2002). Stressors experienced within critical periods of neurodevelopment may exert long-term effects on HPA axis function. Early postnatal adverse experiences such as maternal separation are associated with long-lasting alterations in the basal concentrations of hypothalamic CRH mRNA, hippocampal glucocorticoid receptor mRNA, and median eminence CRH, and with the magnitude of stress-induced CRH, corticosterone, and ACTH release. Adverse early experiences result in alterations in juvenile and adult social behavior, such that animals are more timid, less socially interactive, and more subordinate. Conversely, positive early life experiences during critical developmental periods may have beneficial long-term consequences on the ability to mount adaptive responses to stress or threat. These data indicate that a high degree of plasticity exists in stress-responsive neural systems during the prenatal and early postnatal periods, which may confer either susceptibility or resilience to future stress (see Heim and Nemeroff 2001).

Central Noradrenergic System Function in Stress and PTSD

Exposure to stressful stimuli increases central noradrenergic function, particularly in the LC, hypothalamus, hippocampus, amygdala, and cerebral cortex. The LC is a critical component of the brain's alerting or vigilance system. Rapid activation of the LC-norepinephrine system facilitates the organism's ability to respond effectively in dangerous situations (Charney and Deutch 1996). However, inescapable stress results in a behavioral pattern termed *learned helplessness* (described under Avoidance, Numbing, and Interpersonal Constriction), which includes social withdrawal, reduced food and liquid intake, and reduced aggressiveness. This syndrome has been associated with depletion of norepinephrine, possibly reaching a point where norepinephrine synthesis cannot keep pace with norepinephrine release. Learned helplessness has been suggested as an animal model for PTSD. In humans the helplessness results from involuntary intrusive traumatic memories and perceptions. In contrast with the time-limited syndrome in animals, in PTSD the disorder is persistent and self-perpetuating.

Electrical stimulation of the LC produces a series of behavioral responses similar to those observed in naturally occurring or experimentally induced fear. These behaviors are also elicited by administration of drugs, such as yohimbine and piperoxan, which activate the LC by blocking α_2-adrenergic autoreceptors. Drugs that decrease the function of the LC by interacting with inhibitory opiate (morphine), benzodiazepine (diazepam), and α_2-adrenergic (clonidine) receptors on the LC decrease fearful behavior. The responsiveness of LC neurons to novel stressors is enhanced by previous exposure to stress and may constitute a form of behavioral sensitization (see Increased Arousal), a process by which single or repeated exposures to aversive stimuli or pharmacological agents can increase the neurochemical and behavioral sensitivity to subsequent stressors (reviewed in Charney et al. 1993).

HPA-Axis Function and CRH Release in PTSD

Abnormalities of HPA-axis function have often been reported in PTSD. However, the nature of such abnormalities has been inconsistent. An intriguing finding in the neuroendocrinology of PTSD is the increased cerebrospinal fluid CRH level and normal or reduced cortisol and ACTH concentrations. Two hypotheses propose to explain HPA-axis function in PTSD. The first, the glucocorticoid receptor model, maintains that upregulation of glucocorticoid receptors and increased glucocorticoid receptor sensitivity are the initial impairments in PTSD. These lead to an increased negative feedback of cortisol at the pituitary and adrenal levels (Yehuda 2001) with enhanced CRH production in the extrahypothalamic sites, leading to increased cerebrospinal fluid CRH concentration. Even though CRH is hypersecreted, the glucocorticoid receptor hypersensitivity inhibits cortisol output. Four indirect measures provide support for the assertion that PTSD is related to increased glucocorticoid receptor function.

First, the antiglucocorticoid RU-486 increases cortisol and ACTH levels, indicating that glucocorticoid receptors are involved in the inhibition of the HPA axis. Second, patients with PTSD have greater numbers of lymphocyte glucocorticoid receptors than do healthy control subjects. Third, in response to a dexamethasone suppression test, those with PTSD hypersuppress cortisol. Because dexamethasone selectively binds to glucocorticoid receptors, these data indicate that patients with PTSD evidence a dysfunction in glucocorticoid receptors. Fourth, rodents evidence increased glucocorticoid receptor numbers as well as binding after acute and prolonged stressors. However, other rodent studies have not found these effects on glucocorticoid receptors (Gesing et al. 2001). The major problem with the glucocorticoid receptor model is that 24-hour samplings of cortisol demonstrated that hormone levels in the evening were lower in patients with PTSD than in those of healthy control subjects (Yehuda 2001). Because evening cortisol levels are at trough, high-affinity mineralocorticoid receptors and not glucocorticoid receptors regulate its levels at this time. These data suggest that mineralocorticoid receptors, rather than glucocorticoid receptors, may be involved in the hyperregulation of cortisol.

The second hypothesis, the CRH-mineralocorticoid receptor model, is based on the clinical findings that patients with PTSD secrete high levels of CRH but have normal or low cortisol levels. It is assumed that the CRH levels increase mineralocorticoid receptor numbers, and the mineralocorticoid receptors are responsible for the increased negative feedback of cortisol. The elevated CRH levels may also be related to reduced hippocampal volume, as has been recently shown in animals (Brunson et al. 2001). Support for this proposal comes from preclinical data and animal models of stress. The hippocampus exerts an inhibitory influence on HPA-axis activity (reviewed in Jacobson and Sapolsky 1991). In rodents' brains, glucocorticoid receptors are widely distributed but are particularly dense in the hippocampus and hypothalamic PVN. In higher-order animals such as primates, glucocorticoid receptor distribution may differ. Thus, work by Sanchez et al. (2000) demonstrated low levels of glucocorticoid receptors in hippocampus, although not all studies replicate this finding (Patel et al. 2000). Work by Gesing et al. (2001) demonstrated that a psychological stressor in rats increased mineralocorticoid receptor levels in the hippocampus, neocortex, frontal cortex, and amygdala but not in the hypothalamus. In the same study, pretreatment with a CRH antagonist blocked the stress-related mineralocorticoid receptor increase, whereas infusion of CRH induced a marked increase in hippocampal mineralocorticoid receptors. No effects of stress or CRH were found on glucocorticoid receptors. In another study with rodents, a 15-minute exposure to foot shock evoked increased mineralocorticoid receptor binding capacity in rats (van Dijken et al. 1993). In an investigation with tree shrews, chronic psychosocial stress evoked an increase in mineralocorticoid receptor mRNA content in CA1, CA3, and the dentate of the hippocampus (Meyer et al. 2001). Rats that underwent a stressor showed increased cortisol and ACTH levels following the administration of an mineralocorticoid receptor antagonist relative to nonstressed rats, suggesting that the upregulation of mineralocorticoid receptors in the stressed group is associated with increased inhibitory tone of the HPA axis (Gesing et al. 2001). In humans, the mineralocorticoid receptor antagonist spironolactone leads to increased ACTH and cortisol levels, demonstrating that these receptors exert inhibitory control over the HPA axis. However, increases in ACTH levels are not always statistically significant, suggesting that mineralocorticoid receptor antagonism may increase adrenal sensitivity to ACTH (Young et al. 1998).

Peripheral Noradrenergic Function in PTSD

Considerable evidence also indicates that peripheral noradrenergic function is abnormal in PTSD. Women with PTSD secondary to childhood sexual abuse show increased 24-hour urinary excretion of catecholamines and cortisol. Men (but not women) with PTSD resulting from a motor vehicle accident exhibited elevated urinary levels of epinephrine, norepinephrine, and cortisol 1 month after the accident and still had higher epinephrine levels 5 months later (Hawk et al. 2000). Similarly, maltreated children with PTSD excreted greater amounts of urinary dopamine, norepinephrine, and cortisol over 24 hours than did control subjects, with the urinary catecholamine and cortisol output being positively correlated with the duration of PTSD trauma and the severity of PTSD symptoms (De Bellis et al. 1999). Exposure to traumatic reminders (e.g., combat films or sounds) produces greater increases in plasma, epinephrine, norepinephrine, and cortisol in PTSD patients than in control subjects (Hawk et al. 2000). Geracioti et al. (2001) found that cerebrospinal fluid norepinephrine concentrations are abnormally elevated in PTSD. Platelet α_2-adrenergic receptor density, platelet basal, isoproterenol and forskolin-stimulated cyclic adenosine monophosphate, and basal platelet monoamine oxidase activity were decreased in PTSD. These findings have been hypothesized to reflect compensatory responses to chronically elevated norepinephrine release (for review, see Southwick et al. 1999a).

Subjects with PTSD report that their hyperarousal symptoms and intrusive memories are attenuated by alcohol, benzodiazepines, and opiates—agents known to decrease LC neuronal firing activity—but are exacerbated by cocaine, which increases LC neuronal firing. The risk for abuse of these substances is increased in subjects with PTSD, raising the possibility that such patients are "self-medicating" symptoms with these agents. It remains unclear whether alterations in noradrenergic function play a primary etiological role in the pathogenesis of anxiety disorders or whether they instead reflect secondary, compensatory changes in response to pathology in other systems.

The sensitivity of α_2-adrenergic receptors also appears to be increased in PTSD. Subjects with combat-related PTSD show increased behavioral, chemical, and cardiovascular responses to yohimbine relative to healthy control subjects, and yohimbine administration resulted in altered metabolic activity in the orbital, temporal, parietal, and prefrontal cortices in healthy control subjects relative to PTSD subjects (Southwick et al. 1999a).

Functional Interactions Between Noradrenergic and HPA-CRH Systems

Coordinated interactions between the HPA axis and the noradrenergic systems play a major role in producing an adaptive response to stress. The secretion of CRH increases LC neuronal firing activity, resulting in enhanced norepinephrine release in a variety of cortical and subcortical regions. Conversely, norepinephrine release stimulates CRH secretion in the PVN (the nucleus containing the majority of CRH-synthesizing neurons in the hypothalamus). CRH release in the PVN stimulates ACTH secretion from the pituitary gland and cortisol secretion from the adrenal gland. The rise in plasma cortisol concentration acts through a negative-feedback pathway to decrease both CRH and norepinephrine synthesis at the level of the PVN. Glucocorticoid-mediated inhibition of norepinephrine-induced CRH stimulation may be evident primarily during stress, rather than under resting conditions, as an adaptive response that restrains stress-induced neuroendocrine and cardiovascular effects. Norepinephrine, cortisol, and CRH thus appear tightly linked as a functional system that offers a homeostatic mechanism for responding to stress.

Neurobiology of Emotional Memory

Acquisition of fear-conditioned responses requires an intact central noradrenergic system, which suggests that norepinephrine release plays a critical role in fear learning (Charney and Deutch 1996). For at least some types of emotional learning, memory consolidation depends on noradrenergic stimulation of β- and α_1-adrenergic receptors in the basolateral nucleus of the amygdala (Roozendaal 2000). The activation of norepinephrine release in such models may in turn depend on the effects of stress hormones on noradrenergic neurons. Consolidation of memory may be regulated by interactions between norepinephrine and glucocorticoid secretion. A characteristic feature of PTSD is that memories of the traumatic experience vividly persist for decades and are recalled in response to multiple and diverse stimuli. In experimental animals, alterations of both brain catecholamine and glucocorticoid levels affect the consolidation and retrieval of emotional memories (McGaugh and Roozendaal 2002). Glucocorticoids influence memory storage via activation of glucocorticoid receptors in the hippocampus, whereas the effects of norepinephrine are mediated in part through β-adrenergic receptor stimulation in the amygdala (Roozendaal 2000). In humans, adrenocortical suppression blocks the memory-enhancing effects of amphetamine and epinephrine, and propranolol impairs memory for an emotionally provocative story, but not for an emotionally neutral story (McGaugh 2000). These data suggest that the acute release of glucocorticoids and norepinephrine in response to trauma may modulate the encoding of traumatic memories. It is conceivable that long-term alterations in these systems may account for memory distortions seen in PTSD, such as the memory fragmentation, hypermnesia, and deficits in declarative memory.

Central Benzodiazepine-GABA Receptor System

The benzodiazepine and GABA A receptors form parts of the same macromolecular complex and are functionally coupled and regulate each other in an allosteric manner. Benzodiazepine receptor agonists have anxiolytic effects, whereas inverse agonists have anxiogenic properties. Benzodiazepine binding allosterically changes receptor complex configuration, decreasing or increasing the concentration of GABA required for opening of the chloride channel (Nutt and Malizia 2001). Administration of benzodiazepine receptor inverse agonists induces increases in heart rate, blood pressure, plasma cortisol, and catecholamines similar to those seen in anxiety and stress. These are effectively blocked by administration of benzodiazepine receptor agonists (Nutt and Malizia 2001).

Animals exposed to stress procedures exhibit changes in binding of GABA-benzodiazepine receptor ligands within minutes. These changes in receptor function likely involve neurosteroid allosteric modulation of the receptor complex. Animals exposed to inescapable stress develop a 20%–30% decrease in benzodiazepine receptor binding in the frontal cortex and cerebral cortex, and some studies show reductions in the hippocampus. Increase in ligand binding is more commonly observed after acute stress, and decrease in binding is more frequent after longer-term exposure to stress (reviewed in Deutsch et al. 1994). Stress-induced increase in benzodiazepine receptors is blocked by adrenalectomy and is restored by corticosterone replacement.

Similarly, mRNA levels for hippocampal GABA A receptor subunits were differentially altered by 10 days of corticosterone administration (Orchinik et al. 1995).

Stressors arising early in life may also influence the development of the GABAergic system. In rats, early-life adverse experiences such as maternal separation result in decreased GABA A receptor concentrations in the LC and the nucleus tractus solitarius; reduced benzodiazepine receptor sites in the LC, the nucleus tractus solitarius, the frontal cortex, and the central nucleus and the LA of the amygdala; and reduced mRNA levels for the γ_2 subunit of the GABA A receptor complex in the LC, the nucleus tractus solitarius, and the amygdala (Caldji et al. 2000). The extent to which these developmental responses to early life stress may alter the expression of fear and anxiety in adulthood remains unclear.

Dopaminergic System

Acute stress increases dopamine release and metabolism in specific brain regions. The dopamine innervation of the mPFC appears to be particularly vulnerable to different types of stress. Even brief exposure to stress increases dopamine release and turnover in the prefrontal cortex in the absence of overt changes in other mesotelencephalic dopaminergic innervated regions (Inoue et al. 1994). Low-intensity electric foot shock in rats increases in vivo tyrosine hydroxylase and dopamine turnover in the mPFC but not in the nucleus accumbens or striatum. In contrast, stress of greater intensity enhances dopamine release and turnover in other areas as well (Inoue et al. 1994). Benzodiazepine anxiolytics prevent selective increases in dopamine utilization in the mPFC following mild stress. Anxiogenic benzodiazepine inverse agonists exert an opposite effect. Selective activation of mPFC dopamine neurons can also be induced by intracerebroventricular injection of corticotropin-releasing factor.

Serotoninergic System

Different types of acute stress result in increased serotonin (5-HT) turnover in the mPFC, nucleus accumbens, amygdala, and lateral hypothalamus in experimental animals (see e.g., Inoue et al. 1994). However, exposure to repeated stress within a learned helplessness model resulted in a decrease of 5-HT release in the frontal cortex (possibly reflecting 5-HT depletion by continued release). Pretreatment with benzodiazepine receptor agonists or tricyclic antidepressant drugs prevents the behavioral syndrome of learned helplessness and reduces 5-HT release. Treatment consisting of administration of selective serotonin reuptake inhibitors and infusion of 5-HT into the frontal cortex reverses the behavioral pattern (Petty et al. 1997). Correspondingly, administration of 5-HT receptor antagonists produces behavioral deficits resembling those of learned helplessness (Petty et al. 1997).

Serotonin release may have both anxiogenic and anxiolytic effects. This apparently depends on the region of the forebrain involved and the receptor subtype that is predominantly stimulated. Anxiogenic effects are mediated via 5-HT_{2A} receptor stimulation, whereas stimulation of 5-HT_{1A} receptors is anxiolytic and may even provide resilience to aversive events. Postsynaptic 5-HT_{1A} receptor gene expression is under tonic inhibition by adrenal steroids in the hippocampus, apparently mostly by mineralocorticoid receptors (reviewed in Lopez et al. 1998). 5-HT_{1A} receptor density and mRNA levels decrease in response to stress or cortisol administration and increase after adrenalectomy (Lopez et al. 1998). Stress-induced downregulation of 5-HT_{1A} receptor expression is prevented by adrenalectomy, showing the importance of circulating adrenal steroids in mediating this effect. This regulatory steroid effect is rapid, and 5-HT_{1A} mRNA levels markedly decrease within hours of mineralocorticoid receptor stimulation (Lopez et al. 1998). Conversely, 5-HT_{2A} receptor expression is upregulated during chronic stress and cortisol administration and is downregulated in response to adrenalectomy.

There is increasing evidence for abnormalities in serotoninergic function in subjects with PTSD. Patients with combat-related PTSD had decreased platelet paroxetine binding, suggesting alterations in the 5-HT transporter. Challenge studies probing the serotoninergic system using meta-chlorophenylpiperazine (m-CPP) demonstrated that a subgroup of patients with PTSD develop anxiety and flashbacks on provocation with this agent (for review, see Southwick et al. 1999b). L.L. Davis et al. (1999) used the serotonin-releasing agent and reuptake inhibitor D-fenfluramine in PTSD patients and demonstrated a significantly lower prolactin response compared with that of control subjects, suggesting central serotoninergic dysfunction (Southwick et al. 1999b).

Neuropeptide Y

Neuropeptide Y is a 36–amino acid peptide neurotransmitter that is co-localized with norepinephrine in the LC, amygdala, hippocampus, periaqueductal gray matter, and prefrontal cortex. One of the central and peripheral actions of neuropeptide Y is to inhibit release of the neurotransmitter with which it is co-localized. In numerous preclinical studies, neuropeptide Y has been shown to inhibit the firing rate of LC neurons and to inhibit release of norepinephrine through actions at the presynaptic receptor. Release of neuropeptide Y is related to the intensity and duration of stress. In a recent human study (Morgan et al. 2001), plasma neuropeptide Y levels significantly increased (compared to baseline) in Special Forces soldiers undergoing survival training. This increase in neuropeptide Y was significantly greater than that of non–Special Forces soldiers exposed to the same stressor. A positive correlation was observed between levels of neuropeptide Y and cortisol, whereas a negative correlation was found between dissociation score and neuropeptide Y. In another human study (Rasmusson et al. 2000), subjects with PTSD had lower baseline plasma neuropeptide Y concentrations and blunted yohimbine-stimulated increases in plasma neuropeptide Y compared with healthy control subjects. This suggests that stress-induced decreases in plasma neuropeptide Y may mediate noradrenergic system hyperreactivity and that high levels of neuropeptide Y may offer protection against PTSD.

Cholecystokinin

Cholecystokinin (CCK), a neuropeptide originally discovered in the gastrointestinal tract, is found in high density in the cerebral cortex, amygdala, hippocampus, midbrain periaqueductal gray matter, substantia nigra, and raphe. Its major effect is anxiogenic, and it has important functional interactions with other systems implicated in anxiety and fear (noradrenergic, dopaminergic, benzodiazepine). CCK high-affinity receptors are currently divided into two groups: alimentary (CCK A), and brain (CCK B).

A recent study showed that administration of CCK B receptor antisense significantly suppressed contextual conditioning fear response (i.e., reduced freezing behavior) in rats (Tsutsumi et al. 2001). Administration of CCK B antagonists before exposure to predator smell attenuated subsequent anxious response. The anxiogenic effect of CCK-4, a CCK receptor agonist, is attenuated by administration of the β-adrenergic receptor antagonist propranolol and by long-term treatment with imipramine, which downregulates β-adrenergic receptors. The excitatory anxiogenic effects of CCK and CCK-4 are also anatagonized by benzodiazepines. Studies in healthy human subjects have demonstrated that CCK-4 induces severe anxiety or short-lived panic attacks. This effect is reduced by lorazepam (de Montigny 1989).

In patients with PTSD, induction of anxiety by CCK-4 was accompanied by lower ACTH response than in healthy controls, whereas cortisol concentrations increased equally in both the PTSD and control groups (Kellner et al. 2000). The elevation in cortisol concentrations attenuated more rapidly in the PTSD group than in the control group.

Opioid Peptides

Acute, uncontrollable stress increases secretion of opiate peptides and decreases μ-opiate receptor density. The increase in opioid peptide secretion may contribute to the analgesia observed during emotionally charged conditions and after uncontrollable stress and exposure to fear-conditioned stimuli. This analgesic effect shows evidence of sensitization, because subsequent exposure to less intense shock in rats previously exposed to uncontrollable shock also results in analgesia. Potentially consistent with these data is another finding. Pitman et al. (1990) found that subjects with PTSD showed reduced pain sensitivity compared with veterans without PTSD after exposure to a combat film, an effect that was reversed by the opiate antagonist naloxone. Bremner et al. (1996) reported that during opiate administration, some subjects with combat-related PTSD experienced an attenuation of their hyperarousal symptoms. Because preclinical studies in experimental animals have shown that opiates potently suppress central and peripheral noradrenergic activity, these data appear compatible with the hypothesis that some PTSD symptoms are mediated by noradrenergic hyperactivity (discussed earlier in Peripheral Noradrenergic Function in PTSD). Conversely, during opiate withdrawal, noradrenergic activity increases, and it has been noted that some symptoms of PTSD resemble those of opiate withdrawal (Charney et al. 1993).

Thyrotropin-Releasing Hormone and the Thyroid Axis

Thyroid hormone hypersecretion is associated with anxiety, palpitations, breathing difficulties, and rapid heart rate in individuals recently exposed to traumatic stress. Despite the similarity of these symptoms to a stress response, studies of the relationship between stress and thyroid disease have not been conducted. Although few studies have looked at thyroid function in anxiety disorders, Mason et al. (1994) found elevated levels of triiodothyronine (T_3) in patients with combat-related PTSD, consistent with evidence that stress results in long-lasting increases in thyroid hormone secretion. A recent study showed that T_3 augmentation of selective serotonin reuptake inhibitor treatment may be of therapeutic benefit in patients with PTSD, particularly those with depressive symptoms (Agid et al. 2001).

Arginine Vasopressin

CRH and AVP are the major secretagogues of the HPA-stress system. However, AVP has been studied much less than CRH, and knowledge of the functional activity and pharmacology of AVP and its receptors in the regulation of HPA activity rests largely on studies conducted in rodents. Vasopressin has ACTH-releasing properties when administered alone in humans, a response that may be dependent on the ambient endogenous CRH level. After administration of the combination of AVP and CRH, a much greater ACTH response is seen, and both peptides are required for maximal pituitary adrenal stimulation. The sensitivities of CRH and AVP transcription to glucocorticoid feedback apparently differ, and AVP-stimulated ACTH secretion may be refractory to glucocorticoid feedback. Vasopressinergic regulation of the HPA axis may therefore be critical for sustaining corticotrope responsiveness in the presence of high circulating glucocorticoid levels during chronic stress. It has been proposed that CRH plays a predominantly permissive role in HPA regulation, whereas AVP represents the dynamic mediator of ACTH release.

AVP is primarily released after a variety of stimuli, including increasing plasma osmolality, hypovolemia, hypotension, and hypoglycemia. It has powerful antidiuretic and vasoconstrictor effects. Extrahypothalamic AVP-containing neurons have also been characterized in the rat, notably in the medial amygdala, that innervate limbic structures such as the lateral septum and the ventral hippocampus. In these latter structures, AVP was suggested to act as a neurotransmitter, exerting its action by binding to specific G protein–coupled receptors (i.e., V1a and V1b), which are widely distributed in the central nervous system, including the septum, cortex, and hippocampus. In addition to its role in fluid metabolism regulation, AVP has been implicated in learning and memory processes, pain sensitivity, synchronization of biological rhythms, and the timing and quality of rapid eye movement sleep. In recent years AVP V1 antagonists have exhibited significant anxiolytic and antidepressant effects in various classic animal models (see Griebel et al. 2002 for concise review and series of experiments).

In the only study of AVP in PTSD available in the literature (Maes et al. 1999), increased serum activity of prolyl endopeptidase (an AVP-degrading enzyme) was found in PTSD, suggesting lower AVP levels that would lead to decreased HPA-axis activity. This finding is in accordance with the anxiolytic effect of AVP antagonists described earlier. This finding is of particular interest given the discrepant findings of increased cerebrospinal fluid CRH levels and normal to low cortisol levels reported in PTSD. AVP may therefore play a pivotal role in PTSD and should be studied further in human stress research.

Conclusions

The DSM-IV classification system annulled the traditional distinction between "functional" and "organic" mental disorders. PTSD may be the ultimate example of the futility of this obsolete distinction: an environmentally derived condition displaying a broad range of neurobiological alterations in the brain and periphery alike. In this chapter, we have presented the most salient neurobiological features of PTSD.

Psychiatric research sometimes resembles the Indian parable of the blind men and the elephant—each individual, sensing a different part of the great animal, forms a different concept of the nature of the elephant. However, stress research provides signs of increasing mutual recognition and collaboration. Systematic conceptualization and prospective empirical research linking biological variables, behavior, and cognition are increasingly applied. Genetic, neuroimaging, and neurochemical approaches are combined to provide an integrated biotype of PTSD. Studies investigating the association between heredity, rearing, HPA-CRH function, and stress response are an exceptional example of highly perceptive research and nature-nurture interaction. The magnitude of data collected on PTSD since it was incorporated into psychiatric nosology in 1980 is a tribute to the importance and appeal of this disorder in the eyes of the mental health and neuroscience communities.

References

Agid O, Shalev AY, Lerer B: Triiodothyronine augmentation of selective serotonin reuptake inhibitors in posttraumatic stress disorder. J Clin Psychiatry 62:169–173, 2001

Amat J, Matus-Amat P, Watkins LR, et al: Escapable and inescapable stress differentially alter extracellular levels of 5-HT in the basolateral amygdala of the rat. Brain Res 812:113–120, 1998

American Psychiatric Association: Diagnostic and Statistical Manual of Mental Disorders, 4th Edition. Washington, DC, American Psychiatric Association, 1994

American Psychiatric Association: Diagnostic and Statistical Manual of Mental Disorders, 4th Edition, Text Revision. Washington, DC, American Psychiatric Association, 2000

Bagley J, Moghaddam B: Temporal dynamics of glutamate efflux in the prefrontal cortex and in the hippocampus following repeated stress: effects of pretreatment with saline or diazepam. Neuroscience 77:65–73, 1997

Bonne O, Brandes D, Gilboa A, et al: Longitudinal MRI study of hippocampal volume in trauma survivors with PTSD. Am J Psychiatry 158:1248–1251, 2001

Bouton ME: Context and ambiguity in the extinction of emotional learning: implications for exposure therapy. Behav Res Ther 26:137–149, 1988

Breiter HC, Rauch SL: Functional MRI and the study of OCD: from symptom provocation to cognitive-behavioral probes of corticostriatal systems and the amygdala. Neuroimage 4:S127–S138, 1996

Bremner JD, Southwick SM, Darnell A, et al: Chronic PTSD in Vietnam combat veterans: course of illness and substance abuse. Am J Psychiatry 153:369–375, 1996

Breslau N, Kessler RC: The stressor criterion in DSM-IV posttraumatic stress disorder: an empirical investigation. Biol Psychiatry 50:699–704, 2001

Brewin CR, Andrews B, Rose S, et al: Acute stress disorder and posttraumatic stress disorder in victims of violent crime. Am J Psychiatry 156:360–366, 1999

Bruijnzeel AW, Stam R, Compaan JC, et al: Long-term sensitization of Fos-responsivity in the rat central nervous system after a single stressful experience. Brain Res 819:15–22, 1999

Bruijnzeel AW, Stam R, Compaan JC, et al: Stress-induced sensitization of CRH-ir but not P-CREB-ir responsivity in the rat central nervous system. Brain Res 908:187–196, 2001

Brunson KL, Eghbal-Ahmadi M, Bender R, et al: Long-term, progressive hippocampal cell loss and dysfunction induced by early life administration of corticotropin-releasing hormone reproduce the effects of early life stress. Proc Natl Acad Sci U S A 98:8856–8861, 2001

Buchel C, Morris J, Dolan RJ, et al: Brain systems mediating aversive conditioning: an event-related fMRI study. Neuron 20:947–957, 1998

Caldji C, Francis D, Sharma S, et al: The effects of early rearing environment on the development of GABAA and central benzodiazepine receptor levels and novelty-induced fearfulness in the rat. Neuropsychopharmacology 22:219–229, 2000

Charney DS, Deutch A: A functional neuroanatomy of anxiety and fear: implications for the pathophysiology and treatment of anxiety disorders. Crit Rev Neurobiol 10:419–446, 1996

Charney DS, Deutch AY, Krystal JH, et al: Psychobiologic mechanisms of posttraumatic stress disorder. Arch Gen Psychiatry 50:295–305, 1993

Czeh B, Michaelis T, Watanabe T, et al: Stress-induced changes in cerebral metabolites, hippocampal volume, and cell proliferation are prevented by antidepressant treatment with tianeptine. Proc Natl Acad Sci U S A 98:12796–12801, 2001

Davis LL, Clark DM, Kramer GL, et al: D-Fenfluramine challenge in posttraumatic stress disorder. Biol Psychiatry 45:928–930, 1999

Davis M, Walker DL, Lee Y: Roles of the amygdala and bed nucleus of the stria terminalis in fear and anxiety measured with the acoustic startle reflex. Possible relevance to PTSD. Ann N Y Acad Sci 821:305–331, 1997

De Bellis MD, Baum AS, Birmaher B, et al: A.E. Bennett Research Award. Developmental traumatology. Part I: biological stress systems. Biol Psychiatry 45:1259–1270, 1999

De Bellis MD, Hall J, Boring AM, et al: A pilot longitudinal study of hippocampal volumes in pediatric maltreatment-related posttraumatic stress disorder. Biol Psychiatry 50:305–309, 2001

de Montigny C: Cholecystokinin tetrapeptide induces panic-like attacks in healthy volunteers: preliminary findings. Arch Gen Psychiatry 46:511–517, 1989

Deutsch SI, Rosse RB, Mastropaolo J: Environmental stress-induced functional modification of the central benzodiazepine binding site. Clin Neuropharmacol 17:205–228, 1994

Geracioti TD Jr, Baker DG, Ekhator NN, et al: CSF norepinephrine concentrations in posttraumatic stress disorder. Am J Psychiatry 158:1227–1230, 2001

Gesing A, Bilang-Bleuel A, Droste SK, et al: Psychological stress increases hippocampal mineralocorticoid receptor levels: involvement of corticotropin-releasing hormone. J Neurosci 21:4822–4829, 2001

Griebel G, Simiand J, Serradeil-Le Gal C, et al: Anxiolytic- and antidepressant-like effects of the non-peptide vasopressin V1b receptor antagonist, SSR149415, suggest an innovative approach for the treatment of stress-related disorders. Proc Natl Acad Sci U S A 99:6370–6375, 2002

Hawk LW, Dougall AL, Ursano RJ, et al: Urinary catecholamines and cortisol in recent-onset posttraumatic stress disorder after motor vehicle accidents. Psychosom Med 62:423–434, 2000

Heim C, Nemeroff CB: The role of childhood trauma in the neurobiology of mood and anxiety disorders: preclinical and clinical studies. Biol Psychiatry 49:1023–1039, 2001

Inoue T, Tsuchiya K, Koyama T: Regional changes in dopamine and serotonin activation with various intensity of physical and psychological stress in the rat brain. Pharmacol Biochem Behav 49:911–920, 1994

Jacobson L, Sapolsky R: The role of the hippocampus in feedback regulation of the hypothalamic-pituitary-adrenocortical axis. Endocr Rev 12:118–134, 1991

Kandel ER, Schwartz JH: Molecular biology of learning: modulation of transmitter release. Science 218:433–443, 1982

Kellner M, Wiedemann K, Yassouridis A, et al: Behavioral and endocrine response to cholecystokinin tetrapeptide in patients with posttraumatic stress disorder. Biol Psychiatry 47:107–111, 2000

Korte SM: Corticosteroids in relation to fear, anxiety and psychopathology. Neurosci Biobehav Rev 25:117–142, 2001

LaBar KS, Gatenby JC, Gore JC, et al: Human amygdala activation during conditioned fear acquisition and extinction: a mixed-trial fMRI study. Neuron 20:937–945, 1998

Lanius RA, Williamson PC, Densmore M, et al: Neural correlates of traumatic memories in posttraumatic stress disorder: a functional MRI investigation. Am J Psychiatry 158:1920–1922, 2001

LeDoux JE: Emotion circuits in the brain. Annu Rev Neurosci 23:155–184, 2000

Lee Y, Davis M: Role of the hippocampus, the bed nucleus of the stria terminalis, and the amygdala in the excitatory effect of corticotropin-releasing hormone on the acoustic startle reflex. J Neurosci 17:6434–6446, 1997

Lopez JF, Chalmers DT, Little KY, et al: A.E. Bennett Research Award: regulation of serotonin1A, glucocorticoid, and mineralocorticoid receptor in rat and human hippocampus: implications for the neurobiology of depression. Biol Psychiatry 43:547–573, 1998

Lyons DM, Yang C, Sawyer-Glover AM, et al: Early life stress and inherited variation in monkey hippocampal volumes. Arch Gen Psychiatry 58:1145–1151, 2001

Maes M, Lin AH, Delmeire L, et al: Elevated serum interleukin-6 (IL-6) and IL-6 receptor concentrations in posttraumatic stress disorder following accidental man-made traumatic events. Biol Psychiatry 45:833–839, 1999

Maier SF: Exposure to the stressor environment prevents the temporal dissipation of behavioral depression/learned helplessness. Biol Psychiatry 49:763–773, 2001

Maren S: Neurobiology of Pavlovian fear conditioning. Annu Rev Neurosci 24:897–931, 2001

Mason J, Southwick S, Yehuda R, et al: Elevation of serum-free triiodothyronine, total triiodothyronine, thyroxine-binding globulin, and total thyroxine levels in combat-related posttraumatic stress disorder. Arch Gen Psychiatry 51:629–641, 1994

McEwen BS: Allostasis, allostatic load, and the aging nervous system: role of excitatory amino acids and excitotoxicity. Neurochem Res 25:1219–1231, 2000

McGaugh JL: Memory: a century of consolidation. Science 287:248–251, 2000

McGaugh JL, Roozendaal B: Role of adrenal stress hormones in forming lasting memories in the brain. Curr Opin Neurobiol 12:205–210, 2002

Meyer U, van Kampen M, Isovich E, et al: Chronic psychosocial stress regulates the expression of both GR and MR mRNA in the hippocampal formation of tree shrews. Hippocampus 11:329–336, 2001

Morgan CA 3rd, Wang S, Rasmusson A, et al: Relationship among plasma cortisol, catecholamines, neuropeptide Y, and human performance during exposure to uncontrollable stress. Psychosom Med 63:412–422, 2001

Nutt DJ, Malizia AL: New insights into the role of the GABA(A)-benzodiazepine receptor in psychiatric disorder. Br J Psychiatry 179:390–396, 2001

Orchinik M, Weiland NG, McEwen BS: Chronic exposure to stress levels of corticosterone alters GABAA receptor subunit mRNA levels in rat hippocampus. Brain Res Mol Brain Res 34:29–37, 1995

Orr SP, Roth WT: Psychophysiological assessment: clinical applications for PTSD. J Affect Disord 61:225–240, 2000

Patel PD, Lopez JF, Lyons DM, et al: Glucocorticoid and mineralocorticoid receptor mRNA expression in squirrel monkey brain. J Psychiatr Res 34:383–392, 2000

Petty F, Kramer GL, Wu J: Serotonergic modulation of learned helplessness. Ann N Y Acad Sci 821:538–541, 1997

Phillips RG, LeDoux JE: Differential contribution of amygdala and hippocampus to cued and contextual fear conditioning. Behav Neurosci 106:274–285, 1992

Pitman RK, van der Kolk BA, Orr SP, et al: Naloxone-reversible analgesic response to combat-related stimuli in posttraumatic stress disorder: a pilot study. Arch Gen Psychiatry 47:541–544, 1990

Pitman RK, Shin LM, Rauch SL: Investigating the pathogenesis of posttraumatic stress disorder with neuroimaging. J Clin Psychiatry 62:47–54, 2001

Rasmusson AM, Hauger RL, Morgan CA, et al: Low baseline and yohimbine-stimulated plasma neuropeptide Y (NPY) levels in combat-related PTSD. Biol Psychiatry 47:526–539, 2000

Rasmusson AM, Shi L, Duman R: Downregulation of BDNF mRNA in the hippocampal dentate gyrus after re-exposure to cues previously associated with footshock. Neuropsychopharmacology 27:133–142, 2002

Rauch SL, Whalen PJ, Shin LM, et al: Exaggerated amygdala response to masked facial stimuli in posttraumatic stress disorder: a functional MRI study. Biol Psychiatry 47:769–776, 2000

Reul JM, Holsboer F: Corticotropin-releasing factor receptors 1 and 2 in anxiety and depression. Curr Opin Pharmacol 2:23–33, 2002

Roozendaal B: 1999 Curt P. Richter Award. Glucocorticoids and the regulation of memory consolidation. Psychoneuroendocrinology 25: 213–238, 2000

Sanchez MM, Young LJ, Plotsky PM, et al: Distribution of corticosteroid receptors in the rhesus brain: relative absence of glucocorticoid receptors in the hippocampal formation. J Neurosci 20:4657–4668, 2000

Schuff N, Neylan TC, Lenoci MA, et al: Decreased hippocampal N-acetylaspartate in the absence of atrophy in posttraumatic stress disorder. Biol Psychiatry 50:952–959, 2001

Schulkin J, Gold PW, McEwen BS: Induction of corticotropin-releasing hormone gene expression by glucocorticoids: implications for understanding the states of fear and anxiety and allostatic load. Psychoneuroendocrinology 23:219–243, 1998

Servatius RJ, Ottenweller JE, Bergen MT, et al: Persistent stress-induced sensitization of adrenocortical and startle responses. Physiol Behav 56:945–954, 1994

Shin LM, Whalen PJ, Pitman RK, et al: An fMRI study of anterior cingulate function in posttraumatic stress disorder. Biol Psychiatry 50:932–942, 2001

Southwick SM, Bremner JD, Rasmusson A, et al: Role of norepinephrine in the pathophysiology and treatment of posttraumatic stress disorder. Biol Psychiatry 46:1192–1204, 1999a

Southwick SM, Paige S, Morgan CA 3rd, et al: Neurotransmitter alterations in PTSD: catecholamines and serotonin. Semin Clin Neuropsychiatry 4:242–248, 1999b

Starkman MN, Giordani B, Gebarski SS, et al: Decrease in cortisol reverses human hippocampal atrophy following treatment of Cushing's disease. Biol Psychiatry 46:1595–1602, 1999

Tsutsumi T, Akiyoshi J, Hikichi T, et al: Suppression of conditioned fear by administration of CCKB receptor antisense oligodeoxynucleotide into the lateral ventricle. Pharmacopsychiatry 34:232–237, 2001

van Dijken HH, de Goeij DC, Sutanto W, et al: Short inescapable stress produces long-lasting changes in the brain-pituitary-adrenal axis of adult male rats. Neuroendocrinology 58:57–64, 1993

Villarreal G, King CY: Brain imaging in posttraumatic stress disorder. Semin Clin Neuropsychiatry 6:131–145, 2001

Villarreal G, Hamilton DA, Petropoulos H, et al: Reduced hippocampal volume and total white matter volume in posttraumatic stress disorder. Biol Psychiatry 52:119–125, 2002

Walker DL, Davis M: Double dissociation between the involvement of the bed nucleus of the stria terminalis and the central nucleus of the amygdala in startle increases produced by conditioned versus unconditioned fear. J Neurosci 17:9375–9383, 1997

Yehuda R: Biology of posttraumatic stress disorder. J Clin Psychiatry 62:41–66, 2001

Young EA, Lopez JF, Murphy-Weinberg V, et al: The role of mineralocorticoid receptors in hypothalamic-pituitary-adrenal axis regulation in humans. J Clin Endocrinol Metab 83:3339–3345, 1998

Chapter 2

Psychiatric Epidemiology of Disaster Responses

Carol S. North, M.D., M.P.E.

Although much has been learned about posttraumatic responses among community victims of catastrophic events and combat veterans, less is known about psychiatric effects on survivors of major disasters. Disaster-affected populations are different from other traumatized populations even before experiencing a traumatic event, and their issues after the event may also be expected to have many unique features.

The classic psychiatric disorder associated with traumatic events is posttraumatic stress disorder (PTSD), but human psychological responses to such experiences are far more complex than just one set of symptoms. In addition, there are many aspects of the community, the individuals involved, and the disaster agent itself that contribute to outcomes of the people affected. In this chapter I review the literature on disaster-related PTSD and other psychopathology, psychosocial responses to disasters, and associated factors as an empirical basis to point toward directions for intervention.

Disaster Trauma Theory

The Disaster Agent

Disasters vary in type, being subdivided according to the responsible source. Disaster typology generally includes three major types of disasters: 1) natural disasters described as acts of God, 2) technological accidents resulting from human error, and

3) intentional human acts such as terrorism. Disasters do not necessarily cleanly fit into one category or another, because many events may be considered to consist of contributions from more than one origin (World Health Organization 1991).

Most disaster typology experts agree that in terms of evoking mental health consequences, natural disasters are generally the mildest, technological accidents are intermediate, and willful human acts are the most severe (Baum et al. 1983). However, agreement is not universal, and an important dissenting review and critique of the literature concluded that natural disasters evoke the most severe mental health effects (Rubonis and Bickman 1991). Before more definitive conclusions can be made, studies need to be performed using consistent methodology across several disaster types so that variations in research methods do not create apparent differences in populations affected by different kinds of disasters. Even data collected with methods systematically applied across disaster settings may not be easily disencumbered from the disaster agent type and other characteristics that distinguish it, such as scope and magnitude of the disaster, suddenness of occurrence, unexpectedness, and duration of effects. These aspects may be so inextricably attached to the specific event that they cannot be separated sufficiently for one to draw meaningful conclusions about effects of the disaster type itself.

Other aspects of disasters besides their place in the typology contribute to the development of associated psychopathology. It is intuitive that numbers of fatalities and injuries, amount of property damage, size of the geographic area involved, unexpectedness of the occurrence, duration, and recurrence of the event would be indicators of disaster severity associated with severity of mental health consequences.

The disaster agent is just one aspect of a large set of variables that collectively determine the mental health outcomes of affected populations. Additional factors to consider in predicting disaster mental health effects include preexisting characteristics of the affected population, features unique to the communities involved, individual vulnerabilities and resiliency factors, other life events, and coping strategies.

Preexisting Characteristics of the Affected Population

Disasters are different from other kinds of traumatic events because disasters strike cross-sections of the population randomly without regard to characteristics of the individuals involved (with the exception of floods, which affect lower-income populations living on floodplains and who have relatively high baseline rates of psychopathology). Victims of other kinds of traumatic events in communities and combat veteran populations may have significant preexisting characteristics determining their risk for exposure to traumatic events that are confounded with their postexposure course (Breslau et al. 1998; Helzer et al. 1987). Because the populations may be quite different before as well as after the event, care should be taken before generalizing findings from studies of other kinds of traumatic events to populations affected by disasters.

Characteristics of Affected Communities

Previous studies have noted that conflict, criticism, and other negative responses by communities toward victims can adversely affect postdisaster mental health (Johnes 2000) and that highly supportive communities may experience low rates of postdisaster psychopathology after disaster strikes (North et al. 1989). Small, close-knit communities might be able to provide more comprehensive support for their members, although large urban communities may have more resources to lend to organized support for disaster victims. Community response may be especially influential in the postdisaster adjustment of rescue workers whose mission is to serve the community (Green and Lindy 1994; Hassling 2000).

Other Life Events

Other negative life events following, but not preceding, disasters have been shown to be associated with PTSD (Epstein et al. 1998; Maes et al. 2001; North et al. 1999). However, other life events may be confounded with the effects of disasters that, for example, destroy businesses, resulting in loss of jobs that are included in the negative life event count. Risk for experiencing negative life events may also be confounded with long-standing psychosocial adjustment and personality issues that predate the disaster.

Coping Strategies

Perceptions of the event and personal coping styles may serve as moderators of postdisaster mental health responses. Research studies have demonstrated that avoidant coping strategies are associated with posttraumatic psychopathology, including depression, anxiety, and PTSD (Arata et al. 2000; Gibbs 1989; North et al. 2001). Comparisons of avoidant coping with PTSD symptoms are problematic, however, due to confounding of the avoidant coping with the avoidance symptoms of PTSD. The subgroup of avoidance symptoms that contributes to the diagnosis of PTSD differs from the other PTSD symptom categories of intrusion and hyperarousal. Avoidance symptoms such as going out of one's way to avoid reminders of the event may be considered to represent behavioral choices or coping responses to the event rather than direct effects of the event on emotions and physiological functions such as intrusive memories, insomnia, and difficulty concentrating. Therefore, one must use caution when interpreting associations reported between avoidant coping and PTSD symptoms, because they are inherently confounded by their overlapping content.

Individual Vulnerabilities

Several studies have examined predictors of mental health outcomes following disasters. Predictive variables previously considered have included individual degree of exposure to the disaster, demographic factors, psychiatric history, personality, personal experience and resources, and social support. Gender and predisaster psychiatric history have consistently emerged in separate studies as the most robust predictors of psychiatric difficulties following disasters.

Women are at greater risk for PTSD and major depression, and men are at greater risk for substance abuse after disasters

(Kasl et al. 1981; Lopez-Ibor et al. 1985; Maes et al. 1998; Moore and Friedsam 1959; North et al. 1999, 2002; Robins et al. 1984; Steinglass and Gerrity 1990; Weisaeth 1985). This gender-related pattern is the same as that seen in general and other nondisaster populations (Brady and Randall 1999; Breslau 2002; Bucholz 1999; Fullerton et al. 2001; Pincinelli and Wilkinson 2000). Of the other demographic factors tested in the literature—including age, race, and socioeconomic status—either the findings have been mixed or the evidence has been insufficient to conclude that they have consistent associations with postdisaster outcome.

People with preexisting psychiatric illness are especially likely to experience psychiatric illness after a disaster (Bromet et al. 1982; McFarlane 1989; North et al. 1989, 1994, 1999; Ramsay 1990; Smith et al. 1990; Weisaeth 1985), particularly those who had less exposure to the disaster or who were exposed to milder disasters (Breslau and Davis 1992; Feinstein and Dolan 1991; Hocking 1970; Shore et al. 1986; Smith et al. 1993). Similarly, preexisting personality features have been shown to predict the occurrence of other forms of postdisaster psychopathology such as PTSD (Chen et al. 2001; Liao et al. 2002; Maes et al. 2001; McFarlane 1989; Roy 1982; Southwick et al. 1993).

Social support has been linked to mental health outcomes (Bland et al. 1997; Regehr et al. 2001). Although social support appears to fortify the psychosocial adjustment of men, there is evidence that social networks may be more of a burden than a support for women (Solomon et al. 1987). The problem with trying to understand the role of social support is that it may be as much a function of the individual's psychosocial strength as a determiner of it. Those with good social support networks tend to be those with good adjustment (postdisaster or otherwise), and it is difficult to determine what drives what in the relationship.

Resilience

In the rush to identify psychopathology and deliver treatment for those with postdisaster mental health problems, personal resilience in the face of catastrophic emotional trauma is easily overlooked. Once it is recognized that most people do not develop a psychiatric illness, even those highly exposed to the most catastrophic events (North et al. 1999), the perspective of psychological resilience comes into focus as being relevant for most people involved.

Resiliency factors that protect people from psychiatric disorders and promote recovery from psychiatric illness are the inverse of those associated with psychiatric illness and with chronicity. Therefore, men are recognized as more resilient against PTSD and women as more resilient against the development of substance abuse. In addition, well-developed social support networks, active problem-solving coping patterns, adaptive personalities, and lack of prior psychiatric illness may be considered personal indicators of resilience (Bartone et al. 1989; Gibbs 1989).

In the aftermath of the massive harm and chaos in the wake of disasters, the positive effects that always seem to emerge from great adversity can be lost. Studies have reported that 35%–95% of disaster survivors identify having gained something positive that they would never have experienced otherwise (McMillen 1999; McMillen et al. 1997). If clinicians do not make a point of inquiring about positive aspects of people's experience, they may not learn about this information.

Types of Postdisaster Mental Health Response

Psychiatric Disorder or Subdiagnostic Distress?

One of the most important distinctions to be made in the postdisaster setting is whether diagnosable psychiatric illness is present, or whether the distress is of subdiagnostic proportions. Inflexible conceptual models of postdisaster mental health effects that take a one-size-fits-all approach regard all postdisaster mental health experiences as either normal responses to abnormal events or psychopathology that requires treatment. Alternative views of postdisaster emotional distress as normative suggest the introduction of intervention programs consisting of education, reassurance, and sharing of experiences. Such interventions may be sufficient to help the majority of people who will not develop a psychiatric disorder.

The normative interpretation of postdisaster emotional and psychological experience, however, may overlook individuals with serious psychiatric illness, some of whom may be unhelped or even possibly harmed by interventions designed for the majority with subdiagnostic distress but not psychiatric illness. The position that traumatic experiences cause widespread symptoms consistent with PTSD overestimates the psychiatric impact of the event and unnecessarily pathologizes the distress and emotional upset that represent normative responses to catastrophic events. Therefore, the most effective approach to helping populations affected by disasters is a flexible one that recognizes and provides appropriate psychiatric treatment for psychiatric illness yet also appreciates and responds appropriately to the experience of subdiagnostic distress.

The presence or absence of psychiatric illness determines the type of intervention that is most appropriate for a person's mental health needs. Several different kinds of psychiatric disorders may follow disasters. Of course, the signature diagnosis in disaster settings is PTSD, but other anxiety disorders, major depression, somatization, and substance abuse are other important considerations in the differential diagnosis.

Posttraumatic Stress Disorder

Complexities within the DSM-IV-TR (American Psychiatric Association 2000) diagnostic criteria for PTSD may be easily overlooked in the application of this diagnosis after disasters and in other acutely traumatic settings. PTSD provides one of the rare occasions in psychiatry to render a diagnosis based on a direct causal etiology. The disorder must be causally linked to "direct personal experience of an event that involves actual or threatened death or serious injury" (American Psychiatric Association 2000, p. 463). However, other potentially qualifying experiences for the diagnosis may include vicarious exposure through directly witnessing others in such an event and learning that a loved one was involved in such an event. In addition, the event must evoke a response of fear, helplessness, or horror in the individual.

Once sufficient exposure to a qualifying traumatic event has been determined, requisite numbers of symptoms must be present in three categories: intrusive reexperience (e.g., nightmares of the event, unwanted recollections, flashbacks), avoidance and numbing (avoidance of reminders of the event, inability to feel love, psychogenic amnesia for the event), and hyperarousal (being jumpy and easily startled, sleep disturbance, impaired concentration). The symptoms must arise anew after the event to be counted toward the diagnosis. Merely endorsing the requisite number of symptoms after a qualifying event is still not sufficient for a diagnosis, however. The symptoms must cause significant distress or impairment in functioning, and they must persist for at least a month. Many popular symptom scales used to assess PTSD fail to establish that the symptoms are new after the event, do not determine that the symptoms persist for a month, and fail to document that the symptoms cause significant distress or functional impairment. These shortcomings in measurement result in overestimation of the prevalence of the disorder.

The postdisaster prevalence of PTSD varies widely. PTSD has been described in as few as 2%–4% of survivors of natural disasters such as tornadoes (North et al. 1989), volcanoes (Shore et al. 1986) and mudslides (Canino et al. 1990). In a study of people exposed to dioxin contamination, the prevalence of PTSD was found to be 4%–8% (Smith et al. 1986). Far higher rates of PTSD have also been reported in other studies, including 44% in a study of a dam break and flood (Green et al. 1990), 53% following bushfires, 54% after an airplane crash landing (Sloan 1988), and 50%–100% associated with the crash of an airplane into a shopping mall (Newman and Foreman 1987). The problem with trying to compare the prevalence of PTSD after different kinds of disasters is the lack of uniformity of study methods, especially differences in measurement tools, varied timing of assessment, and inconsistent sampling procedures.

This situation has not improved since the occurrence of the terrorist attacks of September 11, 2001, which were followed by invigorated pursuit of studies of terrorism. Articles published to date about the effects of the attacks have varied in the timing of data collection (from 3–5 days after the event to weeks and months later), have sampled different populations using different methods (such as random-digit telephone sampling or Web-based panel samples selected before the September 11 attacks), have used different instruments of measure, and have deviated from DSM-IV-TR diagnostic criteria in assessing PTSD (such as counting symptoms unrelated to the context of the September 11 events and assessing PTSD symptoms among individuals not exposed to a qualifying stressful event) (Galea et al. 2002; Schlenger et al. 2002; Schuster et al. 2001). Given such differences in multiple aspects of the research methods, meaningful comment on comparison of the stated estimates of PTSD prevalence after September 11—from around 8%–20% in the Manhattan population and 3%–4% in other metropolitan areas (Schuster et al. 2001)—is not possible (Breslau 2001). The data most applicable to estimating the maximum prevalence of PTSD in relation to a terrorist event are the 34% rate of PTSD assessed with a structured diagnostic interview in 182 Oklahoma City bombing survivors who were in the direct path of the bomb blast (North et al. 1999).

Epidemiological research has revealed features of PTSD in postdisaster settings that are worth noting for their relevance to designing mental health policy and interventions. First, PTSD is usually comorbid with another postdisaster psychiatric disorder (McFarlane and Papay 1992; McMillen et al. 2000; North et al. 1994, 1999), a feature consistent with the high comorbidity identified in association with PTSD in more general community settings (Breslau 2001; Breslau et al. 2000). In addition, it seems to be the comorbidity more than just the PTSD that accounts for problems with functioning (North et al. 1999; Sims and Sims 1998). Second, although most people tend to report PTSD symptoms after disasters, the majority of people do not develop PTSD. Third, intrusion and hyperarousal symptoms are highly endorsed but avoidance and numbing symptoms are much less often reported. The avoidance and numbing (PTSD group C) symptoms are strongly predictive of PTSD, and the high sensitivity and specificity of these group C symptom criteria for PTSD suggest that these symptoms may serve as a marker or a gatekeeper for PTSD. By definition according to DSM-IV-TR criteria, 100% of people with PTSD must meet the group C symptom criteria. In the study of direct victims of the Oklahoma City bombing, the group C criteria demonstrated 94% specificity for the full diagnosis of PTSD (North et al. 1999). The group C symptoms were also seen to predict difficulties with functioning, treatment seeking, preexisting psychopathology, postdisaster psychiatric comorbidity, and coping through use of alcohol and drugs (McMillen et al. 2000; North et al. 1999).

Major Depression

The most prevalent comorbid diagnosis with PTSD in postdisaster settings is major depression (David et al. 1996; Green et al. 1992; McFarlane and Papay 1992; North et al. 1994, 1999). Disaster survivors with a history of major depression may be at especially high risk for recurrence or persistence of this disorder after the disaster (North et al. 1989, 1994, 1999).

Substance Abuse

Reported drug or alcohol abuse in postdisaster settings is easily dismissed as "self-medication" of emotional distress and postdisaster psychiatric illness, including major depression and anxiety disorders such as PTSD (Joseph et al. 1993; Pfefferbaum and Doughty 2001). This interpretation of drug or alcohol misuse may be a very attractive explanation because it seems less stigmatizing to be medicating another condition caused by something outside the individual than to have a primary substance use disorder. For postdisaster substance abuse problems to represent self-medication with drugs, however, the onset of the substance abuse must occur after the event rather than predating it. When substance misuse is interpreted as medicating disaster-induced problems, however, it is typically assumed without the benefit of data identifying the temporal sequence of events.

Numerous studies have described increased use of alcohol, tobacco, and other drugs after disasters. Such retrospective reports of increases in substance use have been recorded especially from individuals with preexisting alcohol abuse or other psychiatric difficulties (Joseph et al. 1993; McFarlane 1998; Pfefferbaum and Doughty 2001; Sims and Sims 1998; Smith et al. 1999; Vlahov et al. 2002). After a major earthquake in Japan (Shimizu et al. 2000), alcohol consumption was found to decrease rather than increase, however. No studies have observed postdisaster increases in drug or alcohol consumption to translate into diagnosable substance use disorders.

Reports of increased use of substance abuse treatment after disasters (Marcus 2001) have been inappropriately interpreted as evidence of increased substance abuse after disasters. Increases in substance abuse treatment after disasters could merely represent increased seeking of treatment among those with preexisting problems because of increased availability of treatment, greater awareness of substance abuse, or reduced stigma associated with drug abuse that is attributed to medication of another psychiatric disorder caused by the disaster.

Few studies have actually examined whether new drug or alcohol abuse disorders occur after disasters. These studies have uniformly found the onset of virtually all substance abuse cases to date well before the time of the disaster (David et al. 1996; North et al. 1994, 1999, 2002). Therefore, if use of substances increases after disasters, it does not appear to increase to the point of generating diagnosable cases of substance abuse.

Other Anxiety Disorders

Besides PTSD, which is classified as an anxiety disorder, evidence of other anxiety disorders is sometimes seen after disasters (David et al. 1996; Green et al. 1992), especially panic disorder and phobic disorders (McFarlane and Papay 1992). Compared with major depression, other anxiety disorders studied consistently form a smaller part of the diagnostic comorbidity with PTSD (David et al. 1996; North et al. 1994, 1999, 2002).

Somatization

Although somatization disorder is not described as emerging after disasters (Breslau 1998), a large body of disaster literature has developed pertaining to the phenomenon of medically unexplained complaints, generally known as somatization. Because somatization consists of clinically significant, medically unexplained symptoms, instruments that do not discern medically unexplained from medically based symptoms (Merskey 1995; Ramsay et al.1993; Tennant et al. 1986; Viel et al. 1997) or that fail to distinguish clinically significant somatic complaints from trivial or fleeting physical annoyances do not really measure somatization. Lack of attention to these distinctions will provide data with a mix of medically explained, unexplained, and nonqualifying complaints. Another major shortcoming of such instruments for the measurement of somatization after disasters is their failure to distinguish new somatization symptoms after the disaster from somatization symptoms that existed before the disaster.

It has been well demonstrated that highly somatizing individuals report an array of psychological symptoms without basis in established psychiatric disorders, just as they report multiple medically unexplained somatic symptoms (Lenze et al. 1999). Failure to distinguish this style of symptom overreporting characteristic of highly somatizing individuals in psychiatric and somatic symptom reports may result in inflated estimates of psychopathology in proportion to the representation of highly somatizing individuals in research samples.

In the disaster literature, somatization has been largely assessed with tools that are not designed to discriminate qualifying symptoms, and little effort has been made to control for global endorsing tendencies that artifactitiously associate somatic symptoms with psychological symptoms. Therefore, the degree to which the reported associations between PTSD and somatization (Andreski et al. 1998; Davidson et al. 1991; van der Kolk et al. 1996) are independent of artifacts is unclear. The PTSD/Keane (PK) scale of the Minnesota Multiphasic Personality Inventory has been demonstrated to be incapable of distinguishing between somatization and posttraumatic symptomatology (Wetzel et al. 2000).

Two well-designed studies with prospectively collected predisaster data have examined the occurrence of somatization in disaster-exposed populations compared with that in unexposed populations. A study of mudslides following torrential rains in Puerto Rico (Bravo et al. 1990) found statistically significant yet clinically small increases after the disaster in somatic symptoms among disaster-exposed individuals relative to the nonexposed population. However, the increase in somatization symptoms was considered to be nonspecific and potentially explainable by medical and psychiatric disorders or even by unsanitary conditions following the disaster.

The other study (Robins et al. 1986) examined increases in somatization following dioxin contamination and a series of disasters, including tornadoes, floods, and discovery of radioactive well water. Only one case of somatization disorder was detected—in the unexposed comparison group, with onset before the disaster. Somatization symptoms were not prevalent, and no new somatization symptoms were identified. The study concluded that the disasters had not generated somatization and also that the population was remarkably resilient.

Postdisaster Populations

Different populations may show distinct mental health responses to disasters, depending on their degree of exposure and their preexisting characteristics. People directly in the path of a disaster predominantly develop PTSD. Like the direct victims, families and loved ones of those who died in a disaster also may be candidates for PTSD based on their indirect traumatic exposure to the event through their loved one. They may also be at increased risk for major depression and somatization that may complicate their bereavement (Cowan and Murphy 1985). Also, family members and loved ones of those who have survived direct contact with a disaster may be candidates for PTSD acquired vicariously (American Psychiatric Association 2000). A simplified model for conceptualization of disaster mental health effects is one of concentric rings surrounding the direct disaster experience at the center. The rings represent the degree of exposure to the disaster agent, and as the distance from the center increases, the risk for mental health consequences among the population represented by each ring generally decreases (Shore et al. 1989).

Rescue workers constitute an important segment of the population who are somewhat different from direct victims of disasters. They are selected and self-selected for the type of work involved in disaster recovery efforts, are trained for this work, and have had experience on the job; in addition, they participate in the effort by voluntary choice (Cardeña 1994). Although an extensive body of literature describes mental health effects of disasters on this population, few diagnostic data are available. A study of firefighters involved in rescue and recovery work after the Oklahoma City bombing found a lower incidence of PTSD (13%) compared with that of men who were directly exposed to the bomb blast (23%) (North et al. 2002). The most prevalent diagnosis among the firefighters was alcohol use disorder, identified as actively symptomatic in 24% after the bombing and 47% at some time in their lives. Only 12% had any postdisaster diagnosis that did not involve comorbid alcohol abuse or dependence. Virtually none of the alcohol abuse cases began after the bombing, despite a lag in data collection for new cases to accrue beyond 3 years after the disaster. The finding of such high prevalence of alcohol abuse in this population is not so remarkable given that current alcohol abuse rates of 29% have previously been reported in another study of firefighters not selected for involvement in any disaster (Boxer and Wild 1993).

Outside the direct disaster exposure ring, those with neither personal contact with the disaster agent nor indirect contact via loved ones constitute a very different group diagnostically because they cannot be considered to have PTSD (Abdo et al. 1997). General distress, depression, anxiety, and somatization may be present, however. In the wake of the Oklahoma City bombing, the surrounding communities were considered to have been significantly affected (Pfefferbaum et al. 1999). Following the September 11 terrorist attacks, the entire nation was considered psychologically vulnerable to disaster-related mental health problems (Baker 2002). Studies of these two terrorism events have reported on the prevalence of PTSD symptoms, "symptoms consistent with PTSD," "posttraumatic stress disorder components," "probable PTSD," and "PTSD and subthreshold PTSD" measured by community and household surveys within the surrounding metropolitan areas (Pfefferbaum et al. 1999; Schlenger et al. 2002).

According to the DSM-IV-TR (American Psychiatric Association 2000) definition, people without sufficient exposure to a qualifying traumatic event cannot be considered to have PTSD. Even though hearing the news of the September 11 terrorist attacks was very upsetting, and the public viewed repeated and graphic television images of the planes crashing into the World Trade Center towers, these experiences do not constitute sufficient exposure to a traumatic event required for consideration of the diagnosis. Populations not meeting the requisite exposure criterion cannot logically be considered to have symptoms of a disorder that cannot occur in that population. Therefore, measurement of PTSD symptoms in the surrounding community and particularly in distant metropolitan areas is illogical. This is not to say that these events were not distressing to the general public, as undoubtedly they were. This distress, however, is not the same phenomenon as the psychopathology that is recognized as PTSD among individuals directly exposed to catastrophic events. To group this distress with PTSD not only pathologizes that which constitutes normative response to catastrophic events, but it trivializes the serious nature of psychiatric disease among those who meet the full criteria for PTSD.

Even though the majority of people affected by national-caliber disasters report changes in how they feel and function to survey researchers (Associated Press 2001; North et al. 1999), referring to such experiences among people who are not psychiatrically ill as *symptoms* unnecessarily pathologizes those experiences. Referring to these experiences as *responses* or *reactions* to the disaster would be more appropriate to their categorization as normative experiences (e.g., normal reactions to abnormal events).

The Course of Postdisaster Mental Health Response

Workers in the disaster mental health field have developed a model of stages of experience and recovery from disasters. This model includes a "honeymoon phase," of uplifted spirits and optimism in the setting of community outpouring of sympathy and support, lasting days to weeks that gives way to a later "disillusionment phase," as support runs out and the victims are left to manage on their own, before eventual return to equilibrium over ensuing weeks or months (Raphael and Wilson 1993). These theoretical phases are not fixed and may vary and shift with the setting and within individuals over time. Empirical data have provided useful information about the time course of the development and resolution of postdisaster psychopathology. Studies show that PTSD tends to start early after disasters. Among 182 survivors of the direct bomb blast in the Oklahoma City bombing, 76% of those with PTSD identified its onset as being the same day as the bombing; 94% identified the onset as occurring within the first week; and 98% reported that it began in the first month. No delayed-onset cases occurred after 6 months (North et al. 1999). Similarly, no delayed PTSD was observed in a study of 136 survivors of a mass shooting episode (North et al. 1997).

Even though delayed PTSD is not generally observed after disasters, the *appearance* of delayed PTSD may arise from the well-documented delay in seeking treatment by individuals with PTSD. These cases may be misidentified as delayed-onset cases (Weisaeth 2001). Impressions of delayed PTSD may also occur with assessment of subthreshold cases that typically lack only one or two avoidance or numbing symptoms but later acquire enough symptoms to cross the diagnostic threshold; these can be mistakenly classified as delayed cases in follow-up studies (North et al. 1997).

PTSD in the general population follows a course of considerable chronicity, lasting for a year or longer on average, and for a decade or longer in as many as one-third (Breslau and Davis 1992; Kessler et al. 1995). Less information is available to chart the longitudinal course of psychopathology in disasters, but all PTSD cases identified in Oklahoma City bombing survivors were chronic (lasting at least 3 months) according to the DSM-IV definition (North et al. 1999). In a study of a mass-murder episode in Killeen, Texas, about one-half of the PTSD cases identified within 2 months of the event were still unremitted a year later (North et al. 1997). Few predictors of PTSD recovery have been identified in studies of disaster victims.

Bioterrorism: A Unique Form of Intentional Disaster

Bioterrorism, a subtype of intentional disaster, presents a particularly heinous threat to public security. The features of bioterrorism differ from other forms of terrorism in many ways. First, exposed populations may have no immediate objective indications of contact with the agent, because physical confrontation with biochemical agents may leave no immediate stigmata. Therefore, effects of biological and radiological agents may not reveal themselves until days, weeks, or even years have passed. Because people may not know if they have been exposed, they may be easily influenced by their imaginations or by processes of suggestion that spread through contagion, leading to mass panic. The psychiatric response therefore becomes disarticulated from actual exposure or injury. In bioterrorism, the psychological effects of the attack become part of the mechanism of the disaster agent by interfering with the reparative efforts of medical treatment centers when panicked masses flock to them for treatment, overwhelming the system with their numbers (Norwood et al. 2001).

Because few data are available to help those in the field to fully understand the psychological effects of bioterrorism to guide needed mental health interventions, other types of events such as mass contamination accidents and hysterical epidemics may be most instructive to this underdeveloped area of disaster mental health (Freed et al. 1998; Jones 2000; Kharabsheh et al. 2001). Thus, psychiatric effects of bioterrorism may include not only PTSD, but also elements of somatization (Kawana et al. 2001), mass hysteria, and cancer phobia. Management of the psychosocial and medical effects of this kind of disaster agent extends beyond medical and mental health treatment to include social interventions pertaining to the establishment of careful and accurate communication of risk to minimize panic and restore social roles (Norwood et al. 2001).

Directions for Postdisaster Interventions Based on Epidemiological Research

Much has been learned from disaster epidemiology research that is directly applicable to policy and postdisaster mental health interventions. For example, research on the Oklahoma City bombing was heavily relied on for assessment of mental health intervention needs following the September 11 terrorist attacks in New York City (Norris 2002).

Although each disaster setting is unique, findings from previous studies can be instructive for designing general disaster intervention strategies for future events. First, it should be remembered that after a disaster the majority of people do not become psychiatrically ill, and therefore traditional models of psychiatric treatment fail to constitute appropriate interventions for them. A general principle in contemplating disaster mental health recovery work is that disaster populations can be functionally subdivided into two groups: those who are psychiatrically ill and those with subdiagnostic distress.

Because most PTSD starts very soon after a disaster, screening the population for it may begin early, as soon as people are in a position to be able to start talking about their feelings. (Even though PTSD cannot be diagnosed until symptoms have persisted for a month, in disaster studies individuals with PTSD most often report that their symptoms started very soon after the disaster, providing a window of time for identification of those at risk and the application of preventive measures.) People at highest risk for PTSD include those with the most intense exposure to the disaster agent, people most severely injured in the disaster, the bereaved, and those who sustained other losses such as extensive financial loss and property destruction. Women are at greater risk for PTSD and depression, and men are at greater risk for substance use disorders after disasters.

Previous research suggests that prominent avoidance and numbing responses separate those most likely to have PTSD from those likely to recover on their own. People who have been diagnosed with PTSD or other psychiatric disorders or who are at high risk for them should undergo triage for psychiatric evaluation and management. Although most people report that talking about their experiences is a natural coping mechanism that helps speed healing (North et al. 1999; Smith et al. 1990), people with the prominent avoidance and numbing that is characteristic of PTSD may be unable to tolerate this level of exposure to reminders of the disaster. Therapies that force them to come to terms with it, such as the popular debriefing treatments, may be retraumatizing for them.

An important principle in psychiatric assessment of postdisaster populations is that more often than not PTSD presents with comorbid disorders, especially in mental health treatment settings (North et al. 1999). Therefore, a clinical rule of thumb is not to stop the differential diagnosis there and always to remember to keep looking for other disorders once PTSD is diagnosed. Diagnostic comorbidity in PTSD is a marker for severity of illness and disability and can identify cases needing special attention (North et al. 1999). In addition, the comorbid disorders may be at least as important to the course of recovery and the choice of treatment as the PTSD.

In the process of identifying and assisting people with psychiatric illness after disasters, it is important not to discount the distress of the rest of the people who were involved. Those who are distressed but not psychiatrically ill commonly experience intrusive recollection (nightmares, upsetting memories) and hyperarousal (insomnia, vigilance, jumpiness) but not prominent avoidance and numbing responses. This distressed but not psychiatrically ill group can be reassured that their disturbing symptoms most likely represent normal responses to abnormal events and that they will probably resolve naturally with the passage of time. Recovery in this group may be facilitated through sharing their experiences with trusted others to help with cognitive processing, making meaning, and finding perspective in their lives.

Finally, it is important for workers to remember that a large proportion of PTSD after disasters historically becomes chronic. Just as mental health professionals want to be available to provide assistance early after disasters when psychopathology and anguish are acute, it is equally if not more important for professionals to remain available for this population that is likely to have long-term needs.

References

Abdo T, al-Dorzi H, Itani AR, et al: Earthquakes: health outcomes and implications in Lebanon. J Med Liban 45:197–200, 1997

American Psychiatric Association: Diagnostic and Statistical Manual of Mental Disorders, 4th Edition, Text Revision. Washington, DC, American Psychiatric Association, 2000

Andreski P, Chilcoat H, Breslau N: Post-traumatic stress disorder and somatization symptoms: a prospective study. Psychiatry Res 79:131–138, 1998

Arata CM, Picou JS, Johnson GD, et al: Coping with technological disaster: an application of the conservation of resources model to the Exxon Valdez oil spill. J Trauma Stress 13:23–39, 2000

Associated Press: Attacks leave many depressed, sleepless. Houston Chronicle, September 19, 2001. Available at: http://www.chron.com/cs/CDA/story.hts/special/terror/impact/1055126. Accessed November 14, 2002

Baker DR: A public health approach to the needs of children affected by terrorism. J Am Med Womens Assoc 57:117–118, 2002

Bartone PT, Ursano RJ, Wright KM, et al: The impact of a military air disaster on the health of assistance workers. A prospective study. J Nerv Ment Dis 177:317–328, 1989

Baum A, Fleming R, Davidson LM: Natural disaster and technological catastrophe. Environ Behav 15:333–354, 1983

Bland SH, O'Leary ES, Farinaro E, et al: Social network disturbances and psychological distress following earthquake evacuation. J Nerv Ment Dis 185:188–195, 1997

Boxer PA, Wild D: Psychological distress and alcohol use among fire fighters. Scandinavian Journal of Work and Environmental Health 19:121–125, 1993

Brady KT, Randall CL: Gender differences in substance use disorders. Psychiatr Clin North Am 22:241–252, 1999

Bravo M, Rubio-Stipec M, Canino GJ, et al: The psychological sequelae of disaster stress prospectively and retrospectively evaluated. Am J Community Psychol 18:661–680, 1990

Breslau N: Epidemiology of trauma and posttraumatic stress disorder, in Psychological Trauma. Edited by Yehuda R. Washington, DC, American Psychiatric Press, Washington, DC, 1998, pp 1–29

Breslau N: The epidemiology of posttraumatic stress disorder: what is the extent of the problem? J Clin Psychiatry 62:16–22, 2001

Breslau N: Gender differences in trauma and posttraumatic stress disorder. J Gend Specif Med 5:34–40, 2002

Breslau N, Davis GC: Posttraumatic stress disorder in an urban population of young adults: risk factors for chronicity. Am J Psychiatry 149:671–675, 1992

Breslau N, Kessler RC, Chilcoat HD, et al: Trauma and posttraumatic stress disorder in the community: the 1996 Detroit Area Survey of Trauma. Arch Gen Psychiatry 55:626–632, 1998

Breslau N, Davis GC, Peterson EL, et al: A second look at comorbidity in victims of trauma: the posttraumatic stress disorder-major depression connection. Biol Psychiatry 48:902–909, 2000

Bromet EJ, Parkinson DK, Schulberg HC: Mental health of residents near the Three Mile Island reactor: a comparative study of selected groups. J Prev Psychiatry 1:225–276, 1982

Bucholz K: Nosology and epidemiology of addictive disorders and their comorbidity. Psychiatr Clin North Am 22:221–240, 1999

Canino G, Bravo M, Rubio-Stipec M, et al: The impact of disaster on mental health: prospective and retrospective analyses. Int J Ment Health 19:51–69, 1990

Cardeña E: The domain of dissociation, in Dissociation: Clinical and Theoretical Perspectives. Edited by Lynn S, Rhue J. New York, Guilford, 1994, pp 15–31

Chen CC, Yeh TL, Yang YK, et al: Psychiatric morbidity and posttraumatic symptoms among survivors in the early stage following the 1999 earthquake in Taiwan. Psychiatry Res 105:13–22, 2001

Cowan ME, Murphy DL: Identification of postdisaster bereavement risk predictors. Nurs Res 34:71–75, 1985

David D, Mellman TA, Mendoza LM, et al: Psychiatric morbidity following Hurricane Andrew. J Trauma Stress 9:607–612, 1996

Davidson JRT, Hughes D, Blazer DG, et al: Post-traumatic stress disorder in the community: an epidemiological study. Psychol Med 21:713–721, 1991

Epstein R, Fullerton C, Ursano R: Posttraumatic stress disorder following an air disaster: a prospective study. Am J Psychiatry 155:934–938, 1998

Feinstein A, Dolan R: Predictors of post-traumatic stress disorder following physical trauma: an examination of the stressor criterion. Psychol Med 21:85–91, 1991

Freed D, Bowler R, Fleming I: Post-traumatic stress disorder as a consequence of a toxic spill in northern California. J Appl Soc Psychol 28:264–281, 1998

Fullerton CS, Ursano RJ, Epstein RS, et al: Gender differences in posttraumatic stress disorder after motor vehicle accidents. Am J Psychiatry 158:1486–1491, 2001

Galea S, Ahern J, Resnick H, et al: Psychological sequelae of the September 11 terrorist attacks in New York City. N Engl J Med 346:982–987, 2002

Gibbs MS: Factors in the victim that mediate between disaster and psychopathology: a review. J Trauma Stress 2:489–514, 1989

Green BL, Lindy JD: Post-traumatic stress disorder in victims of disasters. Psychiatr Clin North Am 17:301–309, 1994

Green BL, Lindy JD, Grace MC, et al: Buffalo Creek survivors in the second decade: stability of stress symptoms. Am J Orthopsychiatry 60:43–54, 1990

Green BL, Lindy JD, Grace JC, et al: Chronic posttraumatic stress disorder and diagnostic comorbidity in a disaster sample. J Nerv Ment Dis 180:760–766, 1992

Hassling P: Disaster management and the Goteborg Fire of 1998: when first responders are blamed. Int J Emerg Ment Health 2:267–273, 2000

Helzer JE, Robins LN, McEvoy L: Post-traumatic stress disorder in the general population. Findings of the Epidemiologic Catchment Area survey. N Engl J Med 317:1630–1634, 1987

Hocking F: Psychiatric aspects of extreme environmental stress. Dis Nerv Syst 31:542–545, 1970

Johnes M: Aberfan and the management of trauma. Disasters 24:1–17, 2000

Jones TF: Mass psychogenic illness: role of the individual physician. Am Fam Physician 62:2649–2653, 2655–2656, 2000

Joseph S, Yule W, Williams R, et al: Increased substance use in survivors of the Herald of Free Enterprise disaster. Br J Med Psychol 66:185–191, 1993

Kasl SV, Chisholm RE, Eskenazi B: The impact of the accident at Three Mile Island on the behavior and well-being of nuclear workers. Am J Public Health 71:472–495, 1981

Kawana H, Ishimatsu S, Kanda K: Psycho-physiological effects of the terrorist sarin attack on the Tokyo subway system. Mil Med 166 (suppl 12):23–26, 2001

Kessler RC, Sonnega A, Bromet E, et al: Posttraumatic stress disorder in the National Comorbidity Survey. Arch Gen Psychiatry 52:1048–1060, 1995

Kharabsheh S, Al-Otoum H, Clements J, et al: Mass psychogenic illness following tetanus diphtheria toxoid vaccination in Jordan. Bull World Health Organ 79:764–770, 2001

Lenze EL, Miller A, Munir Z, et al: Psychiatric symptoms endorsed by somatization disorder patients in a psychiatric clinic. Ann Clin Psychiatry 11:73–79, 1999

Liao WC, Lee MB, Lee YJ, et al: Association of psychological distress with psychological factors in rescue workers within two months after a major earthquake. J Formos Med Assoc 101:169–176, 2002

Lopez-Ibor JJ Jr, Soria J, Canas SF, et al: Psychological aspects of the toxic oil syndrome catastrophe. Br J Psychiatry 147:352–365, 1985

Maes M, Delmeire L, Schotte C, et al: Epidemiologic and phenomenological aspects of post-traumatic stress disorder: DSM-III-R diagnosis and diagnostic criteria not validated. Psychiatry Res 81:179–193, 1998

Maes M, Mylle J, Delmeire L, et al: Pre- and post-disaster negative life events in relation to the incidence and severity of post-traumatic stress disorder. Psychiatry Res 105:1–12, 2001

Marcus A: Attacks spark rise in substance abuse treatment; group says stress-related drug, alcohol problems will worsen. HealthScoutNews, December 5, 2001. Available at: http://imedreview.subportal.com/health/Drugs_Alcohol_Tobacco/Drug_Abuse/505078.html. Accessed November 15, 2002

McFarlane AC: The aetiology of post-traumatic morbidity: predisposing, precipitating and perpetuating factors. Br J Psychiatry 154:221–228, 1989

McFarlane AC: Epidemiological evidence about the relationship between PTSD and alcohol abuse: the nature of the association. Addict Behav 23:813–825, 1998

McFarlane AC, Papay P: Multiple diagnoses in posttraumatic stress disorder in the victims of a natural disaster. J Nerv Ment Dis 180:498–504, 1992

McMillen JC: Better for it: how people benefit from adversity. Soc Work 44:455–468, 1999

McMillen JC, Smith EM, Fisher RH: Perceived benefit and mental health after three types of disaster. J Consult Clin Psychiatry 6:733–739, 1997

McMillen JC, North CS, Smith EM: What parts of PTSD are normal: intrusion, avoidance, or arousal? Data from the Northridge, California, earthquake. J Trauma Stress 13:57–75, 2000

Merskey H: The Analysis of Hysteria: Understanding Conversion and Dissociation, 2nd Edition. London, Gaskell, 1995

Moore HE, Friedsam HJ: Reported emotional stress following a disaster. Soc Forces 38:135–138, 1959

Newman JP, Foreman C: The Sun Valley Mall Disaster Study. Paper presented at the 3rd annual meeting of the International Society for Traumatic Stress Studies, Baltimore, MD, October 23, 1987

Norris FH: Psychosocial consequences of disasters. PTSD Research Quarterly 13:1–7, 2002

North CS, Smith EM, McCool RE, et al: Acute post-disaster coping and adjustment. J Trauma Stress 2:353–360, 1989

North CS, Smith EM, Spitznagel EL: Posttraumatic stress disorder in survivors of a mass shooting. Am J Psychiatry 151:82–88, 1994

North CS, Smith EM, Spitznagel EL: One-year follow-up of survivors of a mass shooting. Am J Psychiatry 154:1696–1702, 1997

North CS, Nixon SJ, Shariat S, et al: Psychiatric disorders among survivors of the Oklahoma City bombing. JAMA 282:755–762, 1999

North CS, Spitznagel EL, Smith EM: A prospective study of coping after exposure to a mass murder episode. Ann Clin Psychiatry 13:81–87, 2001

North CS, Tivis L, McMillen JC, et al: Psychiatric disorders in rescue workers of the Oklahoma City bombing. Am J Psychiatry 157:857–859, 2002

Norwood AE, Holloway HC, Ursano RJ: Psychological effects of biological warfare. Mil Med 166:27–28, 2001

Pfefferbaum B, Doughty DE: Increased alcohol use in a treatment sample of Oklahoma City bombing victims. Psychiatry 64:296–303, 2001

Pfefferbaum B, Nixon SJ, Krug RS, et al: Clinical needs assessment of middle and high school students following the 1995 Oklahoma City bombing. Am J Psychiatry 156:1069–1074, 1999

Pincinelli M, Wilkinson G: Gender differences in depression. Critical review. Br J Psychiatry 177:486–492, 2000

Ramsay R: Post-traumatic stress disorder: a new clinical entity? J Psychosom Res 34:355–365, 1990

Ramsay R, Gorst-Unsworth C, Turner S: Psychiatric morbidity in survivors of organised state violence including torture. Br J Psychiatry 162:55–59, 1993

Raphael B, Wilson JP: Theoretical and intervention considerations in working with victims of disaster, in International Handbook of Traumatic Stress Syndromes. Edited by Wilson JP, Raphael B. New York, Plenum 1993, pp 105–117

Regehr C, Hemsworth D, Hill J: Individual predictors of posttraumatic distress: a structural equation model. Can J Psychiatry 46:156–161, 2001

Robins LN, Helzer JE, Weissman MM, et al: Lifetime prevalence of specific psychiatric disorders in three sites. Arch Gen Psychiatry 41:949–958, 1984

Robins LN, Fishbach RL, Smith EM, et al: Impact of disaster on previously assessed mental health, in Disaster Stress Studies: New Methods and Findings. Edited by Shore JH. Washington, DC, American Psychiatric Association, 1986, pp 22–48

Roy W: Risk factors for suicide in psychiatric patients. Arch Gen Psychiatry 39:1089–1095, 1982

Rubonis AV, Bickman L: Psychological impairment in the wake of disaster: the disaster psychopathology relationship. Psychol Bull 109:384–399, 1991

Schlenger WE, Caddell JM, Ebert L, et al: Psychological reactions to terrorist attacks: findings from the National Study of Americans' Reactions to September 11. JAMA 288:581–588, 2002

Schuster MA, Stein BD, Jaycox L, et al: A national survey of stress reactions after the September 11, 2001, terrorist attacks. N Engl J Med 345:1507–1512, 2001

Shimizu S, Aso K, Noda T, et al: Natural disasters and alcohol consumption in a cultural context: the Great Hanshin Earthquake in Japan. Addiction 95:529–536, 2000

Shore JH, Tatum EL, Vollmer WM: The Mount St. Helens stress response syndrome, in Disaster Stress Studies: New Methods and Findings. Edited by Shore JH. Washington, DC, American Psychiatric Press, 1986, pp 77–97

Shore JH, Vollmer WM, Tatum EL: Community patterns of posttraumatic stress disorders. J Nerv Ment Dis 177:681–685, 1989

Sims A, Sims D: The phenomenology of post-traumatic stress disorder. A symptomatic study of 70 victims of psychological trauma. Psychopathology 31:96–112, 1998

Sloan P: Posttraumatic stress in survivors of an airplane crash-landing: a clinical and exploratory research intervention. J Trauma Stress 1:211–229, 1988

Smith DW, Christiansen EH, Vincent R, et al: Population effects of the bombing of Oklahoma City. J Okla State Med Assoc 92:193–198, 1999

Smith EM, Robins LN, Przybeck TR, et al: Psychosocial consequences of a disaster, in Disaster Stress Studies: New Methods and Findings. Edited by Shore JH. Washington, DC, American Psychiatric Association, 1986, pp 49–76

Smith EM, North CS, McCool RE, et al: Acute postdisaster psychiatric disorders: identification of persons at risk. Am J Psychiatry 147:202–206, 1990

Smith EM, North CS, Spitznagel EL: Post-traumatic stress in survivors of three disasters. J Soc Behav Pers 8:353–368, 1993

Solomon SD, Smith EM, Robins LN, et al: Social involvement as a mediator of disaster-induced stress. J Appl Soc Psychol 17:1092–1112, 1987

Southwick SM, Yehuda R, Giller EL: Personality disorders in treatment-seeking combat veterans with posttraumatic stress disorder. Am J Psychiatry 150:1020–1023, 1993

Steinglass P, Gerrity E: Natural disasters and posttraumatic stress disorder: short-term vs. long term recovery in two disaster-affected communities. J Appl Soc Psychol 20:1746–1765, 1990

Tennant C, Goulston K, Dent O: Australian prisoners of war of the Japanese: post-war psychiatric hospitalization and psychological morbidity. Aust N Z J Psychiatry 20:334–340, 1986

van der Kolk BA, Pelcovitz D, Roth S, et al: Dissociation, somatization, and affect regulation: the complexity of adaptation to trauma. Am J Psychiatry 153:83–93, 1996

Viel JF, Curbakova E, Eglite M, et al: Risk factors for long-term mental and psychosomatic distress in Latvian Chernobyl liquidators. Environ Health Perspect 105:1539–1544, 1997

Vlahov D, Galea S, Resnick H, et al: Increased use of cigarettes, alcohol, and marijuana among Manhattan, New York, residents after the September 11th terrorist attacks. Am J Epidemiol 155:988–996, 2002

Weisaeth L: Post-traumatic stress disorder after an industrial disaster, in Psychiatry—The State of the Art. Edited by Pichot P, Berner P, Wolf R, et al. New York, Plenum, 1985, pp 299–307

Weisaeth L: Acute posttraumatic stress: nonacceptance of early intervention. J Clin Psychiatry 62:35–40, 2001

Wetzel RD, Clayton PJ, Cloninger CR, et al: Diagnosis of posttraumatic stress disorder with the MMPI: PK scale scores in somatization disorder. Psychol Rep 87:535–541, 2000

World Health Organization: Psychosocial Guidelines for Preparedness and Intervention in Disaster (document MNH/PSF/91.3). Geneva, World Health Organization, 1991

Chapter 3

Children, Disasters, and the September 11th World Trade Center Attack

Roy Lubit, M.D., Ph.D.
Spencer Eth, M.D.

It is widely believed that children are more resilient than adults. In reality, however, they are more vulnerable than adults to the traumatic events, chaos, and disruptions experienced in disasters. Even in preschoolers, the effects can be serious and persistent (Laor et al. 1997; Pfefferbaum 1997; Vogel and Vernberg 1993; Yule et al. 1999). A better understanding of the myriad ways in which children are vulnerable to and are injured by disasters is needed, as is understanding of the obstacles to delivering mental health services to these children. This knowledge could be used to help limit the development of psychological problems that can adversely affect children and communities for years to come. In this chapter, we review children's responses to disaster and examine the effects on children and the New York City public school system of the September 11th World Trade Center (WTC) attack.

Children's coping skills are inherently less effective than those of adults, resulting in an increased risk of becoming overwhelmed and traumatized in a disaster. Children are particularly susceptible to having their perception of the world and of themselves change as a result of being confronted with the destruction and suffering caused by disasters. As a result, tragedy can interrupt normal developmental lines and cause problems with trust, sense of safety, self-esteem, self-efficacy, interpersonal relations, and moral development. Moreover, the magical thinking of children may produce feelings of responsibility for disasters that can damage self-image. After the WTC disaster, an 11-year-old boy wondered if the twin towers had collapsed and his father had died because he lied about brushing his teeth. Another child, who had been teased about being overweight, feared that her jumping up and down had brought the towers down.

Children's dependency on others increases their vulnerability in a disaster. Research has shown that people with an external locus of control are more vulnerable to trauma than those with an internal locus. Children are also severely affected by the postdisaster crisis state and by the tendency for adults to be preoccupied with rebuilding and therefore less able than usual to provide support. Irritability and stress are common in parents after a disaster and will compound the child's difficult task of rebuilding self-esteem and meaning in the world after the catastrophic collapse of safety. Furthermore, children tend to rely on routine and the structure of their world, and they find changes more difficult than do adults. In a disaster, children often lose their schools, places of worship, and social gathering places.

Another difference between children and adults is that after a few months of mild to moderately impaired functioning, adults can generally return to the status quo ante. Children, however, cannot. Children need to continue to learn social and academic skills to remain in step with their classmates. Depression, anxiety, withdrawal, difficulty concentrating, intrusive recollections, and hyperarousal are likely to interfere with a child's ability to participate in and maximally benefit from social and educational opportunities. A few months of traumatic or grief symptoms that interfere with a child's ability to benefit from these experiences can propel a child off the normal developmental curve. Once a child is out of step with his or her peers and schoolwork, it may not be possible to catch up. As a result, the child may never attain the social, academic, and work competence that would otherwise have been attained. These secondary problems may be more troublesome than the symptoms directly resulting from the trauma.

Huge resources are expended to rebuild the community's infrastructure after a disaster. Schools, roads, hospitals, homes, and businesses are all reconstructed at great expense. The reason all of this is rebuilt is to create a nurturing environment for the people who will continue to live there in the decades to come. Placing children in new homes and schools is of limited benefit if they are filled with despair, their moral development is impaired, they have a foreshortened sense of the future, and their social and academic skills are impaired. Children need help in rebuilding their inner world, as well as their outer world, after a disaster.

What Is a Disaster?

Disasters threaten personal safety, overwhelm defense mechanisms, and disrupt community and family structures. They may also cause mass casualties, destruction of property, and collapse of social networks and daily routines (Gist and Lubin 1999; Ursano et al. 1994; Vogel and Vernberg 1993). The psychological trauma arising from the event and its sequelae can wield a severe blow to a child's sense of security and self, including central organizing fantasies and meaning structures.

A crucial factor in healing after trauma is finding a safe place, which may be impossible in a world surrounded by traumatic reminders. Tens of thousands of people in southern Manhattan fled their homes after September 11, 2001, residing with friends or in hotels without their belongings. Those who stayed in southern Manhattan were subject to foul air and the continuous sight of recovery workers, excavation of ground zero, and massive news coverage. Approximately 5,000 students were transferred to other schools for weeks or months. Places frequented with friends and family were gone forever. Thousands of children lost parents and many more lost someone they knew. Meanwhile, parents suffered from anxiety, irritability, depression, and post-traumatic stress disorder (PTSD). Distressed parents have limited ability to soothe their children and help them cope with their fears of the world and their disillusionment with themselves and adults. These secondary stresses further undermine the support structures needed to heal the emotional wounds resulting from a disaster (Pynoos 1993) and are key factors in the failure of many to recover from the effects trauma (Solomon and Smith 1994).

Disasters affect huge numbers of people. Norris estimates that 6%–7% of Americans are exposed to armed conflict and more numbers to trauma each year (Norris 1988; Ursano et al. 1994). From 1996 through 2001, there were an average of 54 disasters declared by the Federal Emergency Management Agency each year. There were 43 major weather-related disasters in the United States from 1988 to 2001, with losses exceeding $185 billion. Including the damage from earthquakes, the cost of disasters exceeds $300 billion for this period. Around the world, during the last decade, 2 million children died in armed conflict, 1 million were orphaned, 6 million were seriously injured or crippled, 20 million were displaced, and over 10 million have been left with grave psychological injuries (General Assembly 1999). Furthermore, the disruption of war massively increases the number of children who fall prey to sexual exploitation and outright rape.

Human suffering lasts long past the time of rebuilding and extends far beyond those directly affected. PTSD symptoms can last for years, and some children will first develop symptoms years after the event (Sack et al. 1999; Yule et al. 2000). Two years after the bombing in Oklahoma City, 16% of children who lived approximately 100 miles from Oklahoma City reported significant PTSD symptoms related to the event (Pfefferbaum et al. 2000). This is a remarkable finding, because these youths were not directly exposed to the trauma or related to the deceased or injured victims. Two years after the 1972 Buffalo Creek Dam collapse in West Virginia, 37% of children evaluated met "probable" DSM-III-R criteria for PTSD (American Psychiatric Association 1987), and 17 years after the collapse 7% still met criteria (Green et al. 1994). After Hurricane Andrew hit southern Florida and Louisiana in 1992, 86% of children met PTSD criteria at 3 months, 76% met criteria at 7 months, and 69% met criteria at 10 months (LaGreca et al. 1996). Eighteen months after the 1988 Armenian earthquake, 90% of the children living adjacent to the epicenter and 30% of the children from the periphery met the diagnostic criteria for PTSD (Pynoos et al. 1993).

Six weeks after the 1999 Taiwan earthquake, 22% of adolescents ages 12–14 met criteria for PTSD (Hsu et al. 2002). Rates of PTSD and other psychological problems resulting from the disasters were probably affected by the differing developmental levels of the countries and their differing abilities to render support to those affected. The relatively low number in the case of the Taiwan earthquake may be a result of using psychiatric interviews rather than self-reporting forms to establish the diagnosis, the relatively high levels of support the country provided to those affected by the disaster, and cultural factors. After the sinking in 1988 of the cruise ship *Jupiter*, which was carrying a large number of British children on vacation, 50% of child survivors had PTSD shortly after the disaster and 15% had PTSD 5–7 years later (Yule et al. 2000). Pol Pot, head of the Khmer Rouge Communist guerillas, came to power in Cambodia in 1975. During his 4 years in power, approximately 2 million of the country's population of 10 million were killed or died of starvation. Fifteen years after being in Pol Pot's forced labor camps, 24% of youths ages 17–24 met criteria for PTSD (Hubbard et al. 1995). These data actually underestimate the number of children experiencing significant emotional effects, because many children who do not have PTSD develop other anxiety disorders, depression, or substance abuse or show alterations in self-image and beliefs about the world that are detrimental to their emotional development and personality. Functioning can be significantly impaired after a disaster in individuals who do not fulfill DSM-IV-TR criteria for PTSD (Giaconia et al. 1995).

Children with direct exposure to a disaster are not the only ones who are adversely affected (Breton et al. 1993; Pfefferbaum et al. 1999). Nader et al. (1993) found that PTSD symptoms correlated with television exposure as well as with direct exposure (witnessing). Children living outside of New York City with no direct exposure have come to counseling centers with the primary complaint of having symptoms related to September 11. The many thousands of children in New York City who witnessed the destruction of the WTC, thousands more who lost a parent, and millions who lived within a few miles have all found it almost impossible to avoid the multiple replaying of the disaster on television.

Psychiatric Sequelae of Disasters

Disasters have multiple effects on children. They can cause trauma-related psychopathology and neurophysiological changes and can affect emotional development. So that people can provide complete care for traumatized children, each of these sequelae must be understood and addressed. The crucial issue in assessing the impact of trauma and deciding if a child needs treatment is not whether a child fulfills criteria for PTSD or any DSM-IV-TR diagnosis. Rather, the focus is the degree of compromise in social and academic functioning and self-care.

The full impact of a disaster on a child depends on many factors. A child's temperament—threshold of reactivity and strength of reaction—affects susceptibility to trauma (Pynoos 1993; Pynoos et al. 1995). A history of prior trauma increases a child's vulnerability to a disaster. Both parents' level of stress and knowledge of the needs of their children will affect their actions to shield the child from the trauma and soothe the child afterward. The child's psychological strengths and images of the world are also critical. Youngsters with an internal locus of control are significantly less vulnerable than those who feel they are helpless victims of all that befalls them. The meaning the child gives to the event may determine its pathogenic potential (Hendin and Haas 1984). The meaning that an event has for individuals is shaped by their personality, the information they receive, and what adults say to them. After surviving a disaster a child may focus on the suddenness with which disasters can strike and the vulnerability of people to them, or the strength of people to endure and the desire of many to help each other. Separation from parents during or after the disaster (McFarlane et al. 1987; Vogel and Vernberg 1993) and a history of threats to attachment, such as parental separation or illness, increase postdisaster stress (Martini et al. 1990). Children also tend to respond more powerfully if their parents are in distress (Green et al. 1991; Handford et al. 1986; Jones et al. 1994; Laor et al. 1996, 1997; Pynoos et al. 1995; Vogel and Vernberg 1993) or if family communication patterns are disrupted (Bromet et al. 1984). Other important factors include what the child saw (death or grotesque images), whether the child believed that his or her life or that of a loved one was in danger, whether the child or a loved one was injured, how quickly and fully the child was brought to a safe and comfortable place, the unexpectedness and duration of the disaster, whether the disaster was an act of nature or of human cause, whether unanswered screams for help were heard, and whether the child feels guilty over acts of omission or commission (Pynoos 1993; Pynoos et al. 1995).

After a disaster, most children with direct exposure will develop significant psychiatric symptoms, and many will have a diagnosable disorder. The most common symptoms are fear, anhedonia, and attention and learning problems (Anthony et al. 1999). New onset, reactivation, or intensification of specific fears, along with dependent and regressed behavior, is also very common after disasters (Goenjian 1993, Sullivan et al. 1991). Disasters can cause a wide range of anxiety, depressive, and dissociative symptoms as well as behavior disorders. Classic articles described sleep problems; nightmares; trauma-related fears; repetitive trauma-related play; and regression, including clinginess to caretakers, separation anxiety, and loss of previously acquired skills (S.E. Perry et al. 1956; Saylor 1993; Terr 1979; Vogel and Vernberg 1993). Belief that omens predicted the disaster, along with subsequent attention to possible warning signs and a sense of a foreshortened future are also important (Terr 1979). Other common symptoms include intrusive recollections, numbing and withdrawal, hyperarousal, depression, generalized anxiety, panic attacks, problems with concentration, irritability, dysphoria, somatic complaints, and substance abuse (Garrison et al. 1995; LaGreca et al. 1996; Silva et al. 2000). Although PTSD symptoms have a tendency to progressively decrease over time, anxiety and depressive symptoms and behavior problems may well be greater after a few months than in the initial weeks (McFarlane 1987; Vogel and Vernberg 1993). Moreover, the onset of PTSD may be delayed (Sack et al. 1999).

Bereavement is likely if loved ones are killed in the disaster (Pynoos and Nader 1988). Complicated bereavement, a combination of bereavement and trauma, is also common. In complicated bereavement the individual has unusual difficulty successfully completing the bereavement process. This is most likely to arise when death is either violent or sudden, when there are no remains as concrete evidence of death, and when one believes that to cease grieving would be a betrayal of the loved one. Ambivalent relationships, which adolescents often have with parents, also predispose to complicated bereavement.

Children's symptoms vary as a function of age and developmental phase. Young children are not likely to report symptoms of numbing and withdrawal but are likely to have the new onset of aggression or a fear not directly related to the trauma, such as separation anxiety or fear of the dark (Scheeringa et al. 1995). Numbing and withdrawal may appear as regression and loss of previously acquired skills. Intrusive memories in young children are likely to take the form of repetitive, joyless play with traumatic themes, or repetitively drawing pictures of the trauma or acting it out. Generalized anxiety, along with heightened arousal and exaggerated startle reactions, are common. Many children have sleep problems, nightmares without clear content, and somatic complaints. Regression, including loss of skills and increased attachment behavior, is particularly common in young children. Young children develop renewed separation anxiety and new fears, avoid new activities, become aggressive, lose verbal skills and sphincter control, wish to sleep in their parents' bed, whine and have temper tantrums, and night terrors (Bingham and Harmon 1996; Scheeringa et al. 1995).

School-age children may become obsessed with the details of the disaster in an attempt to cope, or they may enter a state of constant anxiety and hyperarousal to prepare for future dangers. Some children withdraw into their own quiet world, whereas others engage in increased aggressive behavior. Concentration problems, distractibility, poor sleep, and nightmares are common in this age group, along with preoccupation with danger and traumatic reminders. Somatic symptoms continue to be a common expression of distress at this age. School-age children may become inconsistent in their behavior, vacillating between being cooperative and argumentative, or from exuberant to inhibited. To avoid painful feelings associated with the disaster, children may avoid social activities and school. They may instead focus their energies on repetitive retelling of the event and on traumatic play. School-age children can engage other children in playing out games that recreate the trauma. Their play and comments may show misunderstandings about what occurred. School-age children can have an inappropriate sense of responsibility for the disaster, reinforced by a tendency toward magical thinking. Time skew entails a child erroneously sequencing events when retelling what happened in a trauma.

As children move into adolescence, their reactions become similar to those of adults. They are likely to have several symptoms of numbing and withdrawal, as well as hyperarousal and actual intrusive memories. To manage their painful feelings, they may retreat from others or throw themselves into various activities. They may become unusually aggressive and oppositional. Adolescents develop a foreshortened view of the future and may precipitously enter into adult activities, leaving school to find a job or marry. They may engage in high-risk behavior—including life-threatening reenactments of the trauma, substance abuse, and unsafe sexual behaviors—to counter the pain of the trauma. They may harbor revenge wishes. Some become depressed and withdraw, and there may be sudden shifts in relationships. Eating disturbances, sleep problems, and nightmares are common. The combination of concentration problems, hyperarousal, dysphoria, and irritability can simulate attention-deficit/hyperactivity disorder, oppositional defiant disorder, conduct disorder, and even bipolar disorder.

Assessing symptomatology and impairment can be difficult, because children frequently report that nothing is wrong either because it is too painful to talk about what happened or because they do not want to upset their parents (Yule and Williams 1990). One school-age child insisted week after week that he had recovered from September 11 but then drew a Mother's Day card of the twin towers on fire. Teachers and parents also tend to underreport the internalizing symptoms of their children (Earls et al. 1988; Korol et al. 1999; Vernberg et al. 1996; Vogel and Vernberg 1993; Yule and Williams 1990). The ability of children to shift from painful affective states to being able to play often leads parents to assume incorrectly that the child has recovered. Studies indicate that counselors and teachers identify fewer than 50% of adolescents with significant, treatable emotional problems. Pediatricians do even more poorly, probably because of their more limited time for interaction, and identify only 25% of those with diagnosable mental disorders (Costello et al. 1988).

Impact of Disasters on Emotional Development

A significant long-term impact of disasters on children is the effect on their emotional and possibly neurobiological development (Cicchetti and Toth 1997; Gaensbauer 1994; B.D. Perry 2001; Pynoos 1993; Pynoos et al. 1995). Both adults and children may experience changes in their views of themselves and others as a result of trauma. Children, however, are far more vulnerable because the basic structures of their personality are still being formed. Their vision of the world as safe or dangerous, helpful or hurtful, predictable or unpredictable, controllable or out of control is in flux. Images of the self as effective or ineffective, brave or cowardly, good or shameful are under revision. Disasters may lead to destruction of children's sense of omnipotence and their abiding faith in their parents' ability to protect them. Disasters also disrupt and distort the networks of life that shape children's development—that is, their family, school, religious organizations, and social organizations. After a disaster, these structures are often unable to provide the usual set of key developmental experiences. Further stressing and compromising children's development after a disaster is the irritability and unavailability of their adult caretakers (Pynoos 1993; Pynoos et al. 1995). The lasting nature of these factors may cause a more profound effect on the life course of greater numbers of children than do PTSD and other psychiatric conditions.

Regulation of Affect and Behavior

The intense negative affective states that arise after disasters can interfere with a child's developing ability to regulate, identify, and express emotions (Pynoos 1993; Pynoos et al. 1995). When

---

feelings are overwhelming, the child cannot reflect, examine, label, express, and control the affect. When this process fails, emotions can produce somatic complaints, psychosomatic problems, or behavioral difficulties. A second way in which disasters interfere with emotional regulation is by leaving children with the memory of intensely painful emotions. Both new situations that remind the child of the disaster and situations that elicit similar affective states can lead to severe distress as the associative pathways in the brain are triggered. As a result, these children experience painful emotions and may not learn to distinguish and control affective states. Children may feel only diffuse excitation. Psychoanalytical perspectives hold that in a traumatic situation, the child's stimulus barrier is overwhelmed (Freud 1920/1962). Regression may occur to a fixation point created by an infantile conflict that the child could not handle and may revive infantile defenses and ways of feeling (Fenichel 1945). Alternatively, the individual could engage in repetition compulsion as a means to gain mastery (Freud 1939/1964).

The intensified startle reactions, hypervigilance, numbing, and withdrawal that often arise after disasters can also interrupt the acquisition of control over feelings. These symptoms interfere with attempts to reflect, express, and manage affect. It is difficult to successfully engage in social and work activities when contending with hypervigilance, startle, numbness, and withdrawal. Without normal developmental experiences, opportunities to habituate to stressful situations and to develop skills to effectively cope will be lost (Pynoos et al. 1995).

The experience of disaster interacts with the child's normal fears of the world, giving credence, solidification, and reinforcement to frightening fantasies. These fears can be reinforced by retaliation fantasies arising from the child's thoughts of taking revenge on a perpetrator. Fear can become a pervasive emotion coloring much of life.

Inhibition of aggressive impulses can be eroded after experiencing a disaster. Seeing violent adults interferes with the development of appropriate impulse control. Moreover, the revenge and retaliation fantasies that often follow disasters can inflame aggressive urges. These fantasies may foster identification with the aggressor and self-righteous belief that one is entitled to behave violently. Moreover, they can lead to preoccupation with aggression, rumination on aggressive images, and a tendency to watch or engage in aggression. For some children, the fear of the destructive power of aggression may promote inhibitions that can interfere with the appropriate use of assertiveness. The resulting inability to be assertive can fuel an image of oneself as a victim and can lead to more intense anger as the individual fails to achieve goals. In time, there may be compensatory outbursts of aggression. Children and adolescents may also turn to substance abuse to manage the painful emotions created by the trauma of a disaster. Revenge fantasies, narcissistic rage, adolescent omnipotence, and access to drugs and weapons may result in an explosive combination that can lead the child to use of violent behavior, adoption of radical ideologies, and association with hate groups (Pynoos et al. 1995; van der Kolk et al. 1991).

Risk taking arises from the convergence of several pathways. As a result of impaired coping skills and intense memories of danger, it is difficult for people who have been traumatized to modulate their perceptions of and reactions to threat. Traumatized individuals may face the unconscious dilemma of being preoccupied with fears of the world or lapsing into a counterphobic denial of danger. Survivor guilt can also predispose to risk taking. Substance abuse, even if motivated by an effort to relieve painful emotions, further curtails appropriate inhibitions.

Core Identity

Disasters markedly affect a child's core identity. Major trauma confronts the individual with unprecedented danger. This novel situation must be integrated into an image of self and the world. Attempts at this integration, however, can significantly undermine existing representations, creating intrapsychic conflict.

Disasters damage self-esteem. The sense of powerlessness in being a victim damages a person's sense of self-efficacy. The tendency of children to blame themselves for trouble, along with magical thinking, can promote a deep sense of guilt or shame.

Moreover, the belief that one did not perform well during a crisis, either due to a harsh superego, objective failure, or someone's unfortunate comment, can result in further damage to self-esteem. This shameful or guilt-ridden self-image can become embedded into the core of the personality and can have tremendous psychodynamic impact on personality development. The individual may become chronically dysthymic, isolative because of embarrassment, or risk prone as a way to disprove the tarnished self-image.

Trauma can also trigger discrepancies in representations of the self, others, and the world and can activate conflicts from earlier developmental periods. It can derail central organizing fantasies (unconscious meaning structures) around which the sense of self is established, leading to developmental arrest (Janoff-Bulman 1985; Ulman and Brothers 1988). The traumatic disruption of early narcissistic fantasies can cause a failure to resolve archaic grandiose fantasies and can lead to a perpetual search to merge with powerful figures (Ulman and Brothers 1988).

The experience of disaster may destroy the child's glorified images of the parents and self. In normal development, children slowly come to terms with the limited abilities of their parents. Premature and sudden collapse of these images may lead to a variety of problems. The child's attachment to parents can be weakened, and the child may search for other figures to identify with. The child may become anxious and may withdraw from social and school activities that are crucial to continued development. The child can also develop a pervasive sense of being defective that constitutes a risk for narcissistic psychopathology, including vulnerability to grandiosity and narcissistic rage (Parson 1988).

Children who experience disasters may develop a foreshortened sense of the future, along with a fear that he or she may die soon from a disaster, a feeling of discontinuity over time, and an inability to project himself of herself into the future (Pynoos et al. 1995). All of these difficulties detract from success in formulating appropriate plans.

Moral development can be significantly affected by experiencing a disaster (Lubit and Billick, in press). Being a victim of a disaster induced by someone who goes unpunished can weaken one's belief in justice, due process, and the legal system. Moreover, intense revenge fantasies can interfere with acceptance and internalization of control of aggressive impulses. Loss of a parent and seeing adults operating under poor emotional control and failing to provide safety further erodes the successful internalization of adult beliefs, abilities, and morality. The weakening of attachment from family and parental stress after a disaster can also affect moral development. Moreover, parents' function as role models, sources of affection, and limit setters may be compromised after a disaster because of their own distress and preoccupations with survival and rebuilding (Garbarino et al. 1991; Pynoos et al. 1995). After a disaster, stress may induce parents to become more rigid and less patient at the same time that the child may become impulsive and disinhibited as a result of the trauma. Faced with an authoritarian parental reaction to behavior the child cannot control, children tend to focus attention on the threatening parent rather than the problems caused by their own behavior. The child may become angry at the world (or at least all authority figures), fail to take any responsibility for events, and develop a "righteously" indignant attitude. Morality becomes external and arbitrary.

Identification with the aggressor, which is also common after trauma, markedly interferes with the development of inhibition of aggressive urges. Furthermore, traumatic anxiety can interfere with the development of prosocial, moral behavior. Children must overcome anxiety to counter the wishes of the group and engage in morally appropriate behavior. Anxiety can block the child's engagement in the social relationships and experiences needed for moral development (Goenjian et al. 1999).

Efforts to master the fear and sense of vulnerability elicited by exposure to a disaster may foster enduring identifications. One possible identification is with rescuers, leading to a long-term preoccupation with saving people (Pynoos et al. 1995; Rachman 1980; Williams 1987). Another possibility is preoccupation with revenge fantasies arising from an identification with the aggressor. Revenge fantasies can also foster a combined identification with both aggressor and victim that can be disorganizing or dangerous (Pynoos 1993; Pynoos et al. 1995).

Relationships and Skills Development

Relationships are negatively affected in several ways by exposure to a disaster. School-age children are likely to participate in driven, joyless reenactments that replace normal fantasy play. Traumatized children may try to convince other children to reenact the trauma with them. They may be irritable, sad, distractible, and aggressive. Their attitude can alienate other children and thereby compromise social development. Moreover, sudden losses of friends through dislocation, death, injury, or tensions among those with differing levels of exposure and symptoms can create a sense of the fragility of relationships and can impede the development of trust and close relationships in the future.

Children exposed to painful and intrusive experiences, either at the hands of perpetrators or rescuers, are at risk for fears about interactions with others. This may lead the child to withdraw socially, to misperceive threats in the environment, and to respond aggressively to neutral or friendly actions. These reactions will markedly impair relationships and foster a vicious cycle of self-fulfilling prophecies and relationship difficulties for years to come.

Anxiety about a broad range of activities compromises the child's ability to engage in social events and develop age-appropriate social skills. Children need a sense of safety and efficacy to venture into the world, explore places, meet strangers, and consolidate these experiences as maturational building blocks. If children are too anxious to go to a friend's house, participate in a school trip, join a sports team, or go to a scout meeting or even to the park, they will lack important social, intellectual, and physical skills that could open the world to them. Failure to acquire skills at the age-appropriate time may propel the child off normal developmental paths, causing lasting deficits. Children who have fallen behind tend to be rejected and are further denied critical life experiences they need to effectively relate to peers. Meanwhile, parents' and teachers' abilities to help children overcome their anxiety and inhibitions may be impaired because of their own traumatic symptoms arising from the disaster.

Impact of Disasters on Families, Schools, and Communities

Much of the impact of disasters on children is a secondary effect deriving from the disruptions of communities. Disasters have a tremendous emotional impact on children's caregivers. Disasters undermine parents' ability to meet their children's emotional needs by traumatizing them and by diverting their attention to rebuilding their homes and addressing pressing financial concerns. Parents and teachers become anxious, depressed, and irritable; increase their use of alcohol; and become unable to maintain historical styles of support and discipline. They may be intolerant of their children's posttraumatic regression, may ignore them, or may flood them with their own anxiety. Traumatized parents and teachers find it very hard to reconstitute the setting necessary for children to heal.

Disasters often destroy the physical structures that children rely on for their daily activities: school, home, places of worship, and places of play. This imposes a serious burden on children, because they are generally unnerved by changes in the usual pattern of daily life. These structures form the basis for all life activities and constitute transitional objects. Therefore, children rely on them for the integrity of their ego function. After a disaster, these normal structures of life are disrupted, destroyed, or converted to traumatic reminders that induce stress reactions. For example, on September 11, 2001, the southern part of Manhattan was in disarray. Children were evacuated from their schools amidst images of burning buildings, smoke, and panic. Furthermore, many children needed to relocate to temporary homes and temporary schools. Their personal belongings and places of play and worship were not available. When they did return home, it was permanently changed. The air quality remained poor in southern Manhattan for months. Traditional places of play no longer existed. The landscape now contained military troops, rescue workers, large vehicles, and poor air, which served as unwelcome traumatic reminders.

Children, and the adults who care for them, can become further stressed and feel unsupported when disasters cause rifts in communities and families. Serious tension and splits can arise among people with different levels of symptoms. Those who are dealing with the disaster by denial and avoidance, along with those not greatly affected, often become impatient and insensitive to those who are more outwardly troubled and who wish to converse about the disaster. Relations can degenerate from lack of understanding or insensitivity to irritation, teasing, and anger. After the WTC disaster, major splits occurred among parents who disagreed about returning children to schools near ground zero. For example, in one elementary school, there were angry confrontations between those who wanted their children to return to the former school several months after September 11 and those who felt that the air quality was not adequate and that returning would be too emotionally troubling for the children. The biggest splits were between the school board officials who insisted that the former schools reopen quickly and the parents who wanted to delay return until everything was back to normal.

There were also threats of divisions between those who had lost loved ones in the disaster and people who had lived in the area and had their community uprooted and severely damaged. Considerable political skill avoided a major battle over whether to place a memorial in Battery Park City. Such a memorial would have drawn countless visitors to the small park used by residents of the area.

Splits in communities can also arise if victims are perceived as weak or defective. Those who experienced injury and property loss can be stigmatized and avoided lest their susceptibility to injury magically contaminate those who were less injured, or remind them of their own vulnerability (Holloway and Fullerton 1994). Stigmatization of victims sometimes occurs because non-victims wish to maintain their vision that the world is predictable and fair so that they can maintain a sense of control (Lerner 1980). Splits can also arise when victims are seen as noble and are acclaimed as heroes, leading some to engage in entitled behavior that may alienate others.

Over time, some victims of disasters become disillusioned and angry with authority figures and aid workers. The emotional and concrete needs of people who survive disasters are so great that it is impossible to fully satisfy them, because life can never be as it was before. In addition, the inevitable confusion that occurs in disasters leads to discontent. The anger of the victim whom rescue personnel are attempting to help is generally very discomforting to those who are working hard to render aid.

The damage disasters do to children, parents, and community structures not only can last for years but also can be passed on to children and have a multigenerational effect (Danieli 1998).

September 11

On September 11, 2001, at 8:48 A.M., hijackers flew a 767 commercial airplane into the north tower of the World Trade Center. Fifteen minutes later, a 757 jet was flown into the south tower. At 9:50 A.M., the south tower collapsed, filling the streets with a black cloud that made it difficult or impossible for people to see clearly or breathe comfortably for blocks around. The north tower collapsed 40 minutes later.

Children's experiences on September 11 and in the months afterward varied considerably depending on what school they were in, their parents' desire and ability to remove them from southern Manhattan, and their parents' and schools' willingness to provide mental health services. Many psychiatrists, psychologists, and other clinicians offered care to children after the disaster. However, political and bureaucratic obstacles, a lack of appreciation of children's needs by many who had control of their lives, and an overwhelming desire to return to normal after the disaster combined to slow the provision of services.

The Evacuation

The planes hit shortly after most children had arrived in school. Many students and teachers in lower Manhattan and parts of Brooklyn were able to see the towers burning. Some watched as people jumped from upper floors to their deaths. Many teachers were in shock, whereas others were resourceful in protecting children from visual exposure. In some schools, the principals were assuming control; in other cases they were nowhere to be seen. Eventually all 8,000 students in the downtown schools were evacuated. Many parents picked up their children, particularly from the elementary schools. Teachers and administrators led an exodus north to safety for the students not collected by their parents. Some high school students reported an orderly retreat, but other teens reported that there was panic and that they were told to run for their lives. Younger children sometimes feared being trampled by older ones. Students and teachers ran and walked 2 miles and then headed in different directions to home, to a friend's house or, in a few instances, to teachers' apartments. Some older students walked several miles to Brooklyn or uptown Manhattan.

Post–September 11 Education

In the following days, life for students varied greatly depending on their home school. Students in Murray Bertram High School and the Chinatown elementary and middle schools returned to their schools within a week. Basic services were limited; there were no telephones and the air quality was poor. Fires continued to burn at ground zero into December. The cleanup effort, which inevitably spewed dust into the air, would continue until the following June. Initially, the foul air prompted the principal of Murray Bertram to consider obtaining gas masks for the children. Many staff members complained of skin and respiratory problems. Children received little attention for their loss of mentors and relatives who worked in the WTC, because only the death of direct caregivers was noted. Fear of another terrorist attack was prominent. Murray Bertram is next to the New York City police headquarters, and many feared it was a terrorist target. Bomb scares led the school to be evacuated several times during the first week back. Later, the children had to face the anthrax alert in Manhattan. A continued sense of threat, such as the one these children faced, has been shown to increase the risk for development of PTSD after traumatic exposure.

Stuyvesant, one of the most exclusive public high schools in the United States, has 3,000 students commuting from across the entire city. After 2 weeks of canceled classes, the school was relocated to Brooklyn Tech High School for an afternoon-only schedule. On October 8, the students returned to Stuyvesant despite the fact that three blocks away fires were burning at ground zero and would continue to burn for another 2 months. Concerns about the air quality persisted for the rest of the school year as barges of debris were loaded near the school's air ducts. The Parent-Teacher Association sued because the air ducts were found to be contaminated. After the students returned to Stuyvesant, the traditional school vital signs were favorable. Attendance was steady, disciplinary actions were down, and grades were up. However, the student body complained that teachers had not given the students any slack after the September 11 disaster.

The students and teachers of two special magnet high schools, Economics and Finance, and Leadership and Public Service, both located within a block from ground zero, merged with other schools. Students and staff of Economics and Finance were moved to Norman Thomas High School near the Empire State Building. Many were uncomfortable with the location because this building was presumed to be a tempting target to terrorists. Air quality concerns were a key issue in the decision by principals and board of education officials about when to return. Advisory reports from scientists varied from assurance that the area was safe to warning that it was inappropriate to return until the cleanup was finished. The air quality was generally considered to be acceptable inside the schools, but outside air, through which students needed to travel each day, was problematic. However, asbestos was found in one stairwell with a grate to the outside, forcing its closure. Students returned to the High School of Leadership and Public Service in mid-January and to Economics and Finance shortly afterward. It should be noted that the Wall Street financial district was by then in full operation again.

The struggle over when to return to the area of ground zero became particularly heated for PS 89. The children spent a month at one school in Greenwich Village and then 5 months sharing another school on the east side of Manhattan. Only 200 of the school's 500 students returned to the original site. Many students were removed by their parents to other schools in Manhattan or outside the city. All of the pre-kindergarten children were disenrolled. Both air quality and having adequate time to psychologically prepare the children to return became prominent political issues that split the parents from the school board and from each other. Parents were very concerned about exposing their children to the air while debris was still being collected and particles were being spewed by dump trucks passing in front of the school. Parents were also concerned that children have adequate time to prepare emotionally for their return. The debate among parents and the school board became very heated, and mental health consultants were asked to support one of the opposing sides. The school board compromised by delaying the relocation beyond its final date. The process of return involved opportunities for children to visit the school in small groups and talk about their feelings. Additional time was provided after the return for discussion, with counselors, of children's emotional reactions. For many children, the return was actually a relief, whereas for others, it led to an increase in trauma-related symptoms.

Researchers at the Columbia University School of Public Health screened a sample of 8,300 students in grades 4–12 throughout New York City public schools during February and March of 2002. One-quarter of these students had significant diagnosable emotional problems. The researchers found that 11% of children had PTSD, 15% had agoraphobia, 9% had panic disorder, 11% had conduct disorder, 12% had separation anxiety, 8% had major depression, 10% had generalized anxiety disorder, and alcohol use was significantly increased in the older children. The base rates are not known because no survey had been done before September 11. Based on surveys in other cities, however, it is fair to state that the rate of 26.5% of students having one of the diagnosable disorders examined is at least twice the usual rate. The prevalence of PTSD, agoraphobia, and panic disorder were several times pre–September 11 base rates. Conduct disorder, separation anxiety, and alcohol use were roughly double pre–September 11 base rates. Major depression and generalized anxiety disorder were roughly 125% of pre–September 11 base rates (Hoven et al. 2002). A variety of factors were noted to increase the risk for PTSD, principally being younger, having been personally exposed or having a family member exposed to the disaster, being female, having experienced a prior trauma, and being Hispanic.

Concerning specific PTSD symptoms, 76% of the children often thought about the WTC event, 45% tried to avoid hearing or thinking about it, 25% had difficulty concentrating, 24% had sleep problems, 18% were not going places or doing things because of reminders of the disaster, 17% had nightmares, 16% avoided people who reminded them of the attack, and 16% did not think about the future. Overall, 87% reported having at least one symptom. By the time of the study, 34% of the children with probable PTSD had sought counseling in school or elsewhere, although the adequacy of the care was not clear. Twenty-two percent sought treatment by professionals outside of school.

Obstacles to Providing Services

September 11, among the most significant disasters in American history, presents an invaluable laboratory for studying what to do, and what not to do, in responding to a large-scale catastrophe. There arose a number of obstacles to providing mental health services to children; such services would have minimized the burden of psychiatric morbidity.

The first problem was the lack of infrastructure for mobilizing and organizing clinicians to see those who would benefit from mental health services. On September 12, large centers for providing comfort and aid to victims' families were established by the city. Innumerable "therapists" offered their services to the hospitals, community-based organizations, and crisis centers that were attempting to help victims and their families. By and large, people were not eager to talk about their feelings. Instead, they were generally exclusively interested in obtaining information about whether their lost loved ones were found. Another problem that arose was vetting the therapists who came forward to offer assistance, because it was impossible to quickly verify the credentials of these therapists. There were further difficulties in assessing their training in or knowledge of trauma. One therapist needed to be escorted by police from a family support center after refusing to listen to officials of the center. Another obstacle was that in the following month, therapists offered only to perform no-fee evaluations rather than the no-fee psychotherapy that was needed.

Second, this disaster underscored the observation that most victims have a limited interest in therapy. People were overwhelmed with taking care of concrete issues and contending with their grief. There seemed to be insufficient time or energy for psychotherapy and little understanding that support from professionals might mobilize the energy and ability needed to focus and perform. Another issue is the incapacitating numbing and withdrawal that leads people to isolate themselves, especially from new people who want to talk about painful topics that people prefer to avoid. Compounding these problems is a pervasive fatigue. One woman said that calling the telephone number to obtain mental health assistance required more energy than she could handle. She needed to have the therapist in the room when she was given information about available services. In addition, many people feel stigmatized by contact with a psychiatrist, sensing that seeing one would indicate that there was something wrong with them or that they were weak. Many highly distressed victims sought therapy only after several months had passed and friends and family members urged the person to get help. During this period, the parents' withdrawal and irritability had significant effects on their children.

A third problem concerned the political and bureaucratic obstacles to the provision of services. It took a long time for government funds to be disbursed. This delayed the process of planning care. In the meantime, many organizations approached schools and offered free programs. These approaches sometimes clashed with existing relationships with service providers. In one case, an agency offering free services did not have experience in delivering child mental health care. Nevertheless, the availability of free services was very tempting to schools. Such competition and jockeying for position among service providers diverted time and resources and caused delays in the schools' decisions about how and when services should be provided.

Once the decision was made regarding mental health consultation, another set of problems arose. Schools often delayed accepting help. Decisions about the implementation of group screening and individual assessment protocols dragged on for many weeks. Schools asked for help and yet delayed accepting it for inconsequential reasons such as a guidance counselor's being on leave. The tendency of principals to want to develop their own arrangements for how therapists would work with their schools absorbed time and resources. Underneath many of these issues may have been discomfort at having outsiders in the schools. There were also cross-professional problems. In one school, a master's-level counselor repeatedly advised therapists with far more experience and training on how to treat the children and told three child psychiatrists that she did not want them in the school. Therapists from outside the board of education who wished to help often did not understand the school system or how to effectively consult and did not always act respectfully or collaboratively. Well-meaning professionals experienced conflict in their efforts to forge collaborative relationships when they had not previously worked together and were stressed by the crisis.

There were 8,000 students evacuated from downtown schools. Rather than screening all of these students quickly, a very sophisticated screening was performed of 8,300 anonymous students distributed throughout the city to assess overall mental health needs in terms of geography and other demographic factors. The board of education objected to rapid targeted screening, because if a student were identified as needing resources, the board of education would be responsible for providing them regardless of whether adequate resources were available. Even some clinicians were worried about the demands imposed by conducting an assessment. In one case, a child psychiatrist objected to children's being asked on a screening instrument about whether they were suicidal, because this finding could require immediate intervention for every child who endorsed it. As a result, schools' referrals of children for treatment involved teachers' and guidance counselors' sending students to mental health workers provided by hospitals and mental health agencies. Referrals tended to be limited to disruptive students, whereas those with internalizing disorders were often ignored. Unfortunately, some of the most troubled students were unable to obtain the assistance they needed, because no medications could be prescribed in the schools, and parents were generally not included in the school-based sessions. Students with more serious problems tended to be referred to medical centers for formal treatment. There was no special funding, however, for those who needed medication. Project Liberty funds, awarded by the Federal Emergency Management Agency, could not be used for those needing psychiatric treatment (rather than crisis counseling) or medication or for children with preexisting psychiatric problems. Many of those who needed help, however, needed assistance because September 11 had resulted in an exacerbation of a prior illness. After 6 months, only a quarter of children with diagnosable disorders had received treatment in school. Only one-third had received treatment anywhere.

Many organizations delivering wide-scale services to victims ignored the needs of children. Businesses that lost many employees in the twin towers set up support groups and offered some counseling through employee assistance programs. Children, however, were largely ignored. Similarly, the fire department offered assistance to the families who had lost loved ones. There were predominantly groups for spouses, parents, and even siblings. Children, however, rarely received services, except in schools.

Lessons to Remember

In the aftermath of a disaster, children, especially those with risk factors, should be screened for problems. Moreover, clinicians skilled in treating traumatized children need to provide adequate mental health services before trauma symptoms interfere with the children's development and produce secondary problems that reinforce the trauma response.

In assessing who needs assistance, the issue is not whether individuals fulfill the criteria for a trauma-related DSM-IV-TR diagnosis, but the degree to which their social and academic functioning is impaired, whether they are improving, and whether the disaster experience has adversely affected their views of themselves and others (Pynoos et al. 1998). Treatment must address current symptoms, developmental delays and skill deficits, and damaged views of the world and oneself. Emotional support and psychoeducation should be given to the parents and teachers who take care of the children so that they will know how to help children and be emotionally stable enough themselves to do so. Adults need to understand the impact of traumatic reminders, be tolerant of time-limited regression and distress, and know how to help children manage their painful feelings.

Accomplishing this mission demands a series of actions to overcome the inevitable obstacles. The first concerns the lack of an adequate infrastructure. Cities need the capability for the assessment of traumatized children and the provision of services. Communities and service organizations must have comprehensive disaster plans in place. Mental health workers need to be trained and credentialed before the disaster occurs. Training of school personnel, pediatricians, and other child workers about all phases of disaster relief is crucial. Widespread mental health screenings of highly exposed populations will be needed, because adults inevitably fail to recognize many youngsters who need help. Moreover, the matter of which mental health organizations will assist which school should be resolved in advance. It is much easier to reach agreement when plans are theoretical. In addition, school systems need to develop mental health services in all schools, because schools are the only place where access to children can be easily arranged. Schools also need close ties to mental health clinics to obtain advice and to be able to refer those with more significant problems.

Community leaders need to understand the importance of mental health services, to make the necessary resources available. Students who are overwhelmed with painful feelings cannot learn. Public officials and opinion leaders need to be helped to understand the crucial role of mental health services in helping children to heal after disasters and return to healthy growth and development. Alliances with public leaders are essential to make resources available and to circumvent bureaucratic roadblocks and political interests.

To persuade people to accept help, the stigma associated with psychotherapy must be lessened. The media attention given to the display of emotions by the New York City police officers and firefighters conveyed the acceptance of sharing feelings of sadness after a disaster. Much more remains to be done. Education of children (and adults) in social and emotional intelligence can facilitate openness to seeking treatment and can promote emotional health by enhancing self-understanding and improving relationships. Yet one must exercise considerable care in selecting a program; few are empirically based and demonstrated to be effective (Cohen 1999, 2001). Best practices focus on developing specific skills (such as problem solving) as well as systemic interventions to create caring, safe, and responsive schools and homes.

Beyond the provision of appropriate mental health care for children and their parents and teachers, the issues of minimizing the trauma and avoiding retraumatization need to be attended to. If at all possible, children need to be close to the primary parenting figure during a disaster. The questions of whether or not to stay in the affected area and how soon to return home are also of great importance. After September 11, many people permanently relocated away from New York City, whereas others left their homes for months. After Cyclone Tracey in Darwin, Australia, parents' reports indicated that children who were evacuated and did not return to Darwin had more school problems than those who either had not been evacuated or had been evacuated and returned (Milne 1977). Najarian et al. (1996), however, found that relocation did not lead to greater symptoms in children after the Armenian earthquake. Permanent moves that markedly interfere with social networks are a problem, at least for adults (Bland et al. 1997). In making a decision about relocation, the overriding concern is that remaining in a dangerous place after a disaster is destructive. Above all else, children need to regain a sense of safety as soon as possible after a disaster. Moreover, recurrent and uncontrolled exposure to traumatic reminders is harmful. Therapeutic exposure to the disaster area should occur before a return to the scene of death and destruction. Once children have had the time and therapeutic exposures necessary to feel reasonably comfortable with their school, community, and home, they can return. Therapeutic exposures include talking about returning, drawing pictures about what they think things will be like, and visiting the sites in small groups with considerable adult support. To stay away indefinitely or permanently may be destructive, because the memories of their homes and schools could then be poisoned, leaving them with unnecessarily painful feelings about their prior lives and with their conditioned fear responses intact.

Another crucial issue in avoiding retraumatization is to limit exposure to the media, because media exposure can promote and exacerbate PTSD symptoms (Kiser et al. 1993; Najarian et al. 1996; Pfefferbaum and Pfefferbaum 1998). The media must face the fact that continual repetitive presentation of graphic pictures of disasters will hold people's attention and improve ratings at the expense of their viewers' mental health. In that regard, obsessive television watching is analogous to an addiction. Parents need to be educated about the impact of media exposure on their children and be encouraged to limit it. Community leaders also need to be careful about how the disaster is commemorated. In New York City, marking an anniversary with low-flying planes and sirens served as a traumatic reminder and was upsetting to thousands of people who lived or worked in lower Manhattan.

Finally, mental health professionals should be remain cognizant that community disasters are not the only sources of trauma to children. Children are traumatized by car accidents, domestic violence, abuse, and crime. These children are no less deserving of help than those who were victims of a terrorist attack, hurricane, or earthquake. School personnel, community leaders, and parents need to be made aware of all of the traumatized children and ensure that the mental health services they need are provided.

References

American Psychiatric Association: Diagnostic and Statistical Manual of Mental Disorders, 3rd Edition, Revised. Washington, DC, American Psychiatric Association, 1987

Anthony JL, Lonigan CJ, Hecht SA: Dimensionality of posttraumatic stress disorder symptoms in children exposed to disaster: results from confirmatory factor analyses. J Abnorm Psychol 108:326–336, 1999

Bingham RD, Harmon RJ: Traumatic stress in infancy and early childhood: expression of distress and developmental issues, in Severe Stress and Mental Disturbance in Children. Edited by Pfeffer CR. Washington, DC, American Psychiatric Press, 1996, pp 499–532

Bland SH, O'Leary ER, Farinaro E, et al: Social network disturbances and psychological distress following earthquake evacuation. J Nerv Ment Dis 185:188–194, 1997

Breton JJ, Valla JP, Lambert ZJ: Industrial disaster and mental health of children and their parents. J Am Acad Child Adolesc Psychiatry 32:438–445, 1993

Bromet EJ, Hough L, Connel M: Mental health of children near the Three Mile Island reactor. Journal of Preventive Psychiatry 2:275–301, 1984

Cicchetti D, Toth SL (ed): Developmental Perspectives on Trauma: Theory, Research, and Intervention, Vol 8. New York, University of Rochester Press, 1997

Cohen J (eds): Educating Minds and Hearts: Social Emotional Learning and the Passage Into Adolescence. New York, Teachers College Press, 1999

Cohen J (ed): Caring Classrooms/Intelligent Schools: The Social Emotional Education of Young Children. New York, Teachers College Press, 2001

Costello EJ, Costello AJ, Edelbrock C, et al: Psychiatric disorders in pediatric primary care: prevalence and risk factors. Arch Gen Psychiatry 45:1107–1116, 1988

Danieli Y (ed): International Handbook of Multigenerational Legacies of Trauma. New York, Plenum, 1998

Earls F, Smith E, Reich W, et al: Investigating psychopathological consequences of a disaster in children: a pilot study incorporating a structured diagnostic interview. J Am Acad Child Adolesc Psychiatry 27:90–95, 1988

Fenichel O: The Psychoanalytic Theory of Neurosis. New York, WW Norton, 1945

Freud S: Beyond the pleasure principle (1920), in The Standard Edition of the Complete Psychological Works of Sigmund Freud, Vol 18. Translated and edited by Strachey J. London, Hogarth Press, 1962, pp 7–64

Freud S: Moses and monotheism (1939), in The Standard Edition of the Complete Psychological Works of Sigmund Freud, Vol 23. Translated and edited by Strachey J. London, Hogarth Press, 1964

Gaensbauer TJ: Therapeutic work with a traumatized toddler. Psychoanal Study Child 49:412–433, 1994

Garbarino J, Kostelny K, Dubrow N: What children can tell us about living in danger. Am Psychol 46:376–383, 1991

Garrison CZ, Bryant ES, Addy CL, et al: Posttraumatic stress disorder in adolescents after Hurricane Andrew. J Am Acad Child Adolesc Psychiatry 34:1193–1201, 1995

General Assembly: Report of the Special Representative of the Secretary General for Children and Armed Conflict froM Colchester Hearings on Children Affected by Armed Conflict of the International Bureau of Children's Rights, October 1, 1999. http://www.ibcr.org/Colchester_Hearings.pdf

Giaconia RM, Reinherz HZ, Silverman A, et al: Traumas and posttraumatic stress disorder in a community population of older adolescents. J Am Acad Child Adolesc Psychiatry 34:1369–1380, 1995

Gist R, Lubin B: Response to Disaster: Psychosocial, Community and Ecological Approaches. Ann Arbor, MI, Braun-Brumfield, 1999

Goenjian A: A mental health relief program in Armenia after the 1988 earthquake: implementation and clinical observations. Br J Psychiatry 163:230–239, 1993

Goenjian AK, Stillwel BN, Steinberg AM, et al: Moral development and psychopathological interference in conscience functioning among adolescents after trauma. J Am Acad Child Adolesc Psychiatry 38:376–384, 1999

Green BL, Korol M, Grace MC, et al: Children and disaster: age, gender, and parental effects on PTSD symptoms. J Am Acad Child Adolesc Psychiatry 30:945–951, 1991

Green BL, Grace MC, Vary MG, et al: Children of disaster in the second decade: a 17-year follow-up of Buffalo Creek survivors. J Am Acad Child Adolesc Psychiatry 33:71–79, 1994

Handford HA, Mayes SD, Mattison RE, et al: Child and parent reaction to the Three Mile Island nuclear accident. J Am Acad Child Adolesc Psychiatry 25:346–356, 1986

Hendin H, Haas AP: The Wounds of War. New York, Basic Books, 1984

Holloway HC, Fullerton CS: The psychology of terror and its aftermath, in Individual and Community Responses to Trauma and Disaster. Edited by Ursano RJ, McCaughey BG, Fullerton CS. Cambridge, Cambridge University Press, 1994, pp 31–45

Hoven CW, Duarte CS, Lucas CP, et al: Effects of the World Trade Center Attack on NYC Public School Students—Initial Report to the New York City Board of Education. New York, Applied Research and Consulting, LLC and Columbia University Mailman School of Public Health and New York State Psychiatric Institute, 2002

Hsu C, Chong M, Yang P, et al: Posttraumatic stress disorder among adolescent earthquake victims in Taiwan. J Am Acad Child Adolesc Psychiatry 41:875–881, 2002

Hubbard J, Realmuto GM, Northwood AK, et al: Comorbidity of psychiatric diagnoses with posttraumatic stress disorder in survivors of childhood trauma. J Am Acad Child Adolesc Psychiatry 34:1167–1173, 1985

Janoff-Bulman R: The aftermath of victimization: rebuilding shattered assumptions, in Trauma and Its Wake. Edited by Figley CR. New York: Brunner/Mazel, 1995, pp 15–35

Jones RT, Ribbe DP, Cunningham P: Psychosocial correlates of fire disaster among children and adolescents. J Trauma Stress 7:117–122, 1994

Kiser L, Heston J, Hickerson S, et al: Anticipatory stress in children and adolescents. Am J Psychiatry 150:87–92, 1993

Korol M, Green BL, Gleser GC: Children's responses to a nuclear waste disaster: PTSD symptoms and outcome prediction. J Am Acad Child Adolesc Psychiatry 38:368–375, 1999

LaGreca AM, Silverman WK, Vernberg EM, et al: Symptoms of posttraumatic stress in children after Hurricane Andrew: a prospective study. J Consult Clin Psychol 64:712–723, 1996

Laor N, Wolmer L, Mayes LC, et al: Israeli preschoolers under Scud missile attacks. Arch Gen Psychiatry 53:416–423, 1996

Laor N, Wolmer L, Mayes LC, et al: Israeli preschool children under Scuds: a 30-month follow-up. J Am Acad Child Adolesc Psychiatry 36:349–356, 1997

Lerner M: Belief in a Just World: A Fundamental Delusion. New York, Plenum, 1980

Lubit R, Billick S: Adolescent moral development, in Textbook of Adolescent Psychiatry. Edited by Rosner R. Washington, DC, American Psychiatric Press (in press)

Martini DR, Ryan C, Nakayama MD, et al: Psychiatric sequelae after traumatic injury. The Pittsburg Regatta accident. J Am Acad Child Adolesc Psychiatry 29:70–75, 1990

McFarlane AC: Posttraumatic phenomena in a longitudinal study of children following a natural disaster. J Am Acad Child Adolesc Psychiatry 26:764–769, 1987

McFarlane AC, Policansky SK, Irwin C: A longitudinal study of the psychological morbidity in children due to natural disaster: Psychol Med 17:727–738, 1987

Milne G: Cyclone Tracey II: the effects on Darwin children. Aust Psychol 12:55–62, 1977

Nader KO, Pynoos RS, Fairbanks LA, et al: A preliminary study of PTSD and grief among children of Kuwait following the Gulf crisis. Br J Clin Psychol 32:407–416, 1993

Najarian LM, Goenjian AK, Pelcovitz D, et al: Relocation after a disaster. J Am Acad Child Adolesc Psychiatry 35:374–383, 1996

Norris FH: Toward establishing a database for the prospective study of traumatic stress. Paper presented at the National Institute of Mental Health Workshop: Traumatic Stress: Defining Terms and Instruments, Uniformed Services University of the Health Sciences, Bethesda, MD, 1988

Parson ER: Post-traumatic self-disorder (PTsfD): theoretical and practical considerations in psychotherapy of Vietnam veterans, in Human Adaptation to Extreme Stress: From the Holocaust to Vietnam. Edited by Wilson JP, Harel Z, Kahana B. New York, Plenum, 1988, pp 245–279

Perry BD: The neurodevelopmental impact of violence in childhood, in Textbook of Child and Adolescent Forensic Psychiatry. Edited by Schetky D, Benedek E. Washington, DC, American Psychiatric Press, 2001, pp 221–238

Perry SE, Silber E, Bloch DA: The child and his family in disaster: a study of the 1953 Vicksburg tornado. Washington, DC, National Academy of Sciences, National Research Counsel, 1956

Pfefferbaum B: Posttraumatic stress disorder in children: a review of the past 10 years. J Am Acad Child Adolesc Psychiatry 36:1503–1511, 1997

Pfefferbaum B, Pfefferbaum R: Contagion in stress: an infectious disease model for posttraumatic stress in children. Child Adolesc Psychiatr Clin N Am 7:183–194, 1998

Pfefferbaum B, Nixon SJ, Krug RS, et al: Clinical needs assessment of middle and high school students following the 1995 Oklahoma City bombing. Am J Psychiatry 156:1069–1074, 1999

Pfefferbaum B, Seale TW, McDonald NB, et al: Posttraumatic stress two years after the Oklahoma City bombing in youths geographically distant from the explosion. Psychiatry 63:358–370, 2000

Pynoos RS: Traumatic stress and developmental psychopathology, in American Psychiatric Press Review of Psychiatry, Vol 12. Edited by Oldham JM, Riba MB, Tasman A. Washington, DC, American Psychiatric Press, 1993, pp 205–238

Pynoos RS, Nader K: Psychological first aid and treatment approach to children exposed to community violence: research implications. J Trauma Stress 1:445–473, 1988

Pynoos RS, Goenjian A, Tashjian M, et al: Post-traumatic stress reactions in children after the 1988 Armenian earthquake. Br J Psychiatry 163:239–247, 1993

Pynoos RS, Steinberg AM, Wraith R: A developmental model of childhood traumatic stress, in Developmental Psychopathology: Risk, Disorder, and Adaptation, Vol 2. Edited by Cicchetti D, Cohen DJ. New York, Wiley, 1995, pp 72–95

Pynoos RS, Goenjian AK, Steinberg AM: A public mental health approach to the postdisaster treatment of children and adolescents. Child Adolesc Psychiatr Clin N Am 7:195–227, 1998

Rachman S: Emotional processing. Behav Res Ther 18:51–60, 1980

Sack WH, Him C, Dickason D: Twelve-year follow-up study of Khmer youths who suffered massive war trauma as children. J Am Acad Child Adolesc Psychiatry 38:1173–1179, 1999

Saylor C (ed): Children and Disasters. New York, Plenum, 1993

Scheeringa MS, Zeanah CH, Drell MJ, et al: Two approaches to the diagnosis of posttraumatic stress disorder in infancy and early childhood. J Am Acad Child Adolesc Psychiatry 34:191–200, 1995

Silva RR, Alpert M, Munox DM, et al: Stress and vulnerability to posttraumatic stress disorder in children and adolescents Am J Psychiatry 157:1229–1235, 2000

Solomon SD, Smith EM: Social support and perceived control as moderators of responses to dioxin and flood exposure, in Individual and Community Responses to Trauma and Disasters: The Structure of Human Chaos. Edited by Ursano R, McCaughey B, Fullerton C. Cambridge, Cambridge University Press, 1994, pp 179–200

Sullivan MA, Saylor CF, Foster KY: Post-hurricane adjustment of preschoolers and their families. Adv Behav Res Ther 13:163–171, 1991

Terr L: Children of Chowchilla: a study of psychic trauma. Psychoanal Study Child 34:547–623, 1979

Ulman RB, Brothers D: The Shattered Self: A Psychoanalytic Study of Trauma. Hillsdale, NJ, Analytic Press, 1988

Ursano RJ, McCaughey BG, Fullerton CS (eds): Individual and Community Responses to Trauma and Disaster. Cambridge, Cambridge University Press, 1994

van der Kolk BA, Perry JC, Herman JL: Childhood origins of self-destructive behavior. Am J Psychiatry 148:1665–1671, 1991

Vernberg EM, La Greca AM, Silverman WEK, et al: Prediction of posttraumatic stress symptoms in children after Hurricane Andrew. J Abnorm Psychol 105:237–248, 1996

Vogel JM, Vernberg EM: Children's psychological responses to disasters. J Clin Child Psychol 22:464–484, 1993

Williams W: Reconstruction of an early seduction and its aftereffects. J Am Psychoanal Assoc 35:145–163, 1987

Yule W, Williams RM: Post-traumatic stress reactions in children. J Trauma Stress 3:279–295, 1990

Yule W, Perrin S, Smith P: Post-traumatic stress reactions in children and adolescents, in Posttraumatic Stress Disorders: Concepts and Therapy. Edited by Yule W. Chichester, United Kingdom, Wiley, 1999, pp 25–50

Yule W, Bolton D, Udwin O, et al: The long-term psychological effects of a disaster experienced in adolescence, I: the incidence and course of PTSD. J Child Psychol Psychiatry 41:503–511, 2000

Chapter 4

Early Intervention for Trauma-Related Problems

Patricia J. Watson, Ph.D.
Matthew J. Friedman, M.D., Ph.D.
Laura E. Gibson, Ph.D.
Josef I. Ruzek, Ph.D.
Fran H. Norris, Ph.D.
Elspeth Cameron Ritchie, M.D.

The study of early intervention following exposure to traumatic stress has accelerated greatly in the past decade, with the goal of finding ways to prevent the psychopathology and deterioration in functioning that are so often associated with exposure to severe stress. Unfortunately, the evidence for effective early interventions, particularly after mass trauma, remains very limited. This matter was addressed by experts from around the world at a recent consensus conference on psychological interventions after mass violence. Conference attendees concluded that current evidence from randomized controlled trials (RCTs) does not permit definitive confirmation or refutation of the effectiveness of any early psychological intervention after major incidents. In addition, the empirical literature suggests that psychological debriefing, a common intervention during the acute posttraumatic period, does not ameliorate acute posttraumatic distress, does not prevent subsequent psychopathology (Bisson et al. 2000), and

A number of federal agencies were represented, including U.S. Department of Health and Human Services, U.S. Department of Defense, U.S. Department of Veterans Affairs, U.S. Department of Justice, and American Red Cross.

may even exacerbate subsequent symptoms of posttraumatic stress disorder (PTSD) (Rose et al. 2000).

In this chapter, we review the available evidence and present areas of research concerning effective early intervention following exposure to traumatic stress, especially with respect to mass casualties. We begin by reviewing the literature on the psychological impact of disasters, with special attention to risk and protective factors. This is followed by a detailed review of research on a variety of early interventions after trauma, including psychological debriefing, cognitive-behavioral therapy, treatment for traumatic grief, interventions for children, and pharmacotherapy.

Empirical Literature on the Effects of Disasters

We begin by summarizing the substantial literature published over the past 20 years on the psychological effects of disasters. More details can be found in a recent article (Norris et al. 2002) that reviewed current research findings from 160 samples of people who had experienced 102 different disasters. Three sample-level predictors were examined in this review: disaster type, sample type, and disaster location. With regard to type of disaster, mass violence was by far the most disturbing kind of disaster studied. Whereas 67% of samples exposed to mass violence were severely impaired, 39% of samples exposed to technological disasters and 34% of samples exposed to natural disasters were severely impaired (meaning that at least 25% of the sample met study criteria for psychopathology). For instance, after the Oklahoma City bombing, almost half of survivors directly exposed to the blast reported developing problems with anxiety, depression, and alcohol, and more than one-third reported PTSD. Predictors of PTSD, anxiety, and depression included more severe exposure, female gender, and having a psychiatric disorder before the bombing (North et al. 1999). As for sample type, school-age youths were the most likely—and rescue and recovery workers the least likely—to demonstrate severe impairment: 62% of the school-age samples experienced severe impairment, compared with 39% of the adult survivor samples and 7% of the rescue/recovery samples. Disaster location had an even stronger effect on outcomes than either disaster type or sample type: 78% of the samples from developing countries met criteria for severe impairment, compared with 25% of the United States samples and 48% of the samples from other developed countries.

The general rule with regard to the course of postdisaster distress was for the sample to improve as time passed. These effects were not always linear; many victims and survivors reported initial improvement, followed by a period of stabilization or worsening, followed by later improvement. Symptoms usually peaked in the first year and were less prevalent thereafter, leaving only a minority of communities and individuals substantially impaired. The first anniversary was generally associated with intensification of distress and increased use of mental health services. Levels of symptoms in the early phases of disaster recovery were good predictors of symptoms in later phases. Delayed onsets of psychological disorders were rare.

Norris and colleagues (2002) concluded that when 1) injuries and deaths are rare, 2) the destruction or loss of property is confined relative to the size and resources of the surrounding community, 3) social support systems remain intact and function well, and 4) the event does not take on more symbolic meanings of human neglect or maliciousness, then disasters seem to have minimal adverse mental health consequences at the population level beyond those associated with transient stress reactions. In contrast, the authors concluded that risk for impairment was greatest when at least two of the following factors were present: 1) extreme and widespread damage to property; 2) serious and ongoing financial problems for the community; 3) human carelessness or, especially, human intent causing the disaster; or 4) high prevalence of trauma in the form of injuries, threat to life, and loss of life. Many of the studies reviewed by Norris and colleagues examined individual-level risk and protective factors within these samples. Of these, the factors that most consistently increased risk for adverse outcomes included 1) severe exposure to the disaster, especially injury, threat to life, and extreme loss; 2) living in a highly disrupted or traumatized community;

3) female gender; 4) age in the middle years of 40–60; 5) little previous experience or training relevant to coping with the disaster; 6) membership in an ethnic minority group; 7) poverty or low socioeconomic status; 8) the presence of children in the home; 9) for women, the presence of a spouse, especially if he is significantly distressed; 10) psychiatric history; 11) secondary stress; and 12) weak or deteriorating psychosocial resources.

The protection afforded by psychological and social resources has important implications for interventions. For instance, self-efficacy, mastery, perceived control, self-esteem, hope, and optimism all are related positively, strongly, and consistently to mental health, whereas avoidance coping and blame seem to be consistently problematic. Beliefs about capabilities for coping prove to be far more important than specific ways of coping. The size, vitality, and closeness of the survivor's social network is also related strongly and consistently to positive mental health outcomes. Disaster survivors who believe that they are cared for by others and that help will be available, if needed, in the near future fare better psychologically than disaster survivors who believe they are unloved and alone.

The greater the amount of global resource loss, the greater the psychological distress. Several studies have found such measures to be the strongest predictors of symptom outcomes. Psychological resources, such as optimistic biases and perceived control, have occasionally been found to decline after disasters. Social resources appear to be especially vulnerable to the effects of disasters. Declines in social support account for a large share of victims' subsequent declines in mental health. Potential social supporters may themselves have become victims. Families and friends are relied on more often, and with greater comfort, than outsiders or professional sources of support. Sustaining helping activities may be more difficult than mobilizing them. With the passage of time, attentive media, helping organizations, and outside resources disappear. Fatigue, irritability, and scarcity of resources increase the potential for interpersonal conflict and social isolation.

Such deterioration is unlikely when postdisaster support provisions are adequate, equitably distributed, and sufficiently lasting to address survivors' needs. Public education about how much support can reasonably be provided by their social network is an important way to help people calibrate their expectation to what can reasonably be delivered. Professionals and outsiders are important sources of assistance when the level of need is high, but they cannot supplant natural helping networks. It is always best to keep people in their natural social setting if they must be relocated. When networks have been severely disrupted or destroyed, however, it is desirable to foster social activities and help develop new communities. Examples include group meetings, in which survivors collectively plan how to rebuild their community, identify and discuss local problems, work together toward achievable goals, canvass the community to learn of others' needs, and emotionally share their individual and collective losses. Collective grieving, including memorial services, helps people express solidarity and facilitates unity and collective action.

Family-focused interventions are also very important. People are usually most comfortable seeking and receiving help from family members, yet family members can also be a significant source of strain and conflict. Building and sustaining support at the family level is crucial, such as encouraging families to talk together about their experiences, losses, and feelings. Families should also be encouraged to resume normal activities to the extent possible and to handle conflict appropriately so as to minimize negative encounters caused by the strain, fatigue, and irritability that often follow trauma.

Large-scale individual-focused interventions often are not targeted to those in need and therefore can be costly and unnecessary. They should be reserved for those persons who are most distressed, who had weak psychological and social resources to begin with, or who suffered particularly dire resource losses. Because people in greatest need of such services may be least likely to seek them, outreach is essential. Sprang (2000) reported that after a disaster, many of those closest to the event do not believe that they need help and will not seek out services, despite reporting significant emotional distress. Survivors often report feeling that they are better off than those more affected, and they generally believe that acknowledgment of distress is an indication of weakness of some sort; they have a preference for seeking informal support from family and friends (Sprang 2000). Some people are more likely to accept help for problems in living than to accept help for mental health problems. Outreach and education of family members and friends become crucial under these circumstances.

Key Components of Early Intervention

International experts who attended the aforementioned Mass Violence and Early Intervention conference (National Institute of Mental Health 2002) endorsed nine key components of early intervention. These components, outlined as follows, are multifaceted and overlap in time; are provided by diverse individuals, organizations, and professionals; and create a framework within which recovery from traumatization can be maximized. Operationally defining each component of early intervention in this way should facilitate research on the delivery, phasing, and specific effectiveness of each component for both immediate and long-term recovery.

Provision for Basic Needs

Essential for mental health are the meeting of basic needs for safety, security, and survival, such as food and shelter; orientation to the disaster and recovery efforts; facilitating communication with family, friends and community; and reducing ongoing environmental threat.

Psychological First Aid

Basic strategies to reduce psychological distress include orientation to the disaster and recovery efforts, reduction of physiological arousal, mobilization of support for those who are most distressed, facilitation of reunion with loved ones and keeping families together, providing education about available resources and coping strategies, and using effective risk communication techniques.

Needs Assessment

A systematic assessment of the current status of individuals, groups, and the overall affected community is important. Included in the assessment should be an evaluation of whether survivors' needs are being adequately addressed, assessment of the characteristics of the recovery environment, and consideration of what additional interventions and resources are required.

Monitoring of the Rescue and Recovery Environment

Those most affected by the incident are observed and monitored for potential behavioral and physical health sequelae. The environment is monitored for ongoing stressors or toxins, services that are being provided, and media coverage and rumors.

Outreach and Information Dissemination

After disasters and incidents of mass violence, services are provided in the many environments where survivors can be found (sometimes referred to as *therapy by walking around*). Established community structures are used to provide information and support. Information is disseminated via distribution of fliers and referral to Web sites, which can also provide on-line support. The media are provided with materials (e.g., interviews, releases, and programs) to help increase knowledge about trauma and recovery.

Technical Assistance, Consultation, and Training

Organizations, leaders, responders, and caregivers are supported via the dissemination of knowledge, consultation, and training, so that they can improve their capacity to provide what is needed to reestablish community structure, foster family recovery and resilience, and safeguard the community.

Fostering Resilience and Recovery

Resources are provided to improve social interactions, coping skills, risk assessment, and self-assessment and referral. This also includes group and family interventions, fostering natural social support, looking after the bereaved, and repairing the community and organizational fabric.

Triage

Mental health personnel assess survivors, identify vulnerable, high-risk individuals and groups, and provide referral and emergency hospitalization when indicated.

Treatment

Mental health personnel seek to reduce symptoms and improve functioning via education; individual, family, and group psychotherapy; pharmacotherapy; spiritual/existential support; and short-term or long-term hospitalization.

General Recommendations

Participants at the mass violence consensus conference unanimously endorsed the following recommendations for early intervention:

- Interventions should be tailored to address individual, community, and cultural needs and characteristics.
- A sensible working principle in the immediate postincident phase is to expect normal recovery.
- The presumption of clinically significant disorder in the early postincident phase is inappropriate, except for those with pre-existing conditions.
- Interventions should promote normal recovery, resilience, and personal growth.
- Mental health personnel must be integrated into the major incident or disaster management teams and should help coordinate the provision of service so that mental health is an integrated element of comprehensive disaster management plans.
- Mental health expertise can help guide the implementation of interventions to maximize positive mental health outcome.

Good practice in early intervention takes into account the special needs of those who have previously experienced enduring mental health problems, those who are disabled, and other high-risk groups that are disadvantaged so as to be less able to cope with unfolding situations.

Adverse outcomes to be targeted or prevented by early interventions include acute stress disorder (ASD), PTSD, depression, complicated bereavement reactions, substance use disorders, poor physical health, fear, anxiety, physiological arousal, somatization, anger control problems, functional disability, and arrest or regression of childhood developmental progression (National Institute of Mental Health 2002).

Psychological Debriefing

Debriefing means different things to different people. In its broadest sense, it is the process of describing an event or activity. It has become popularized as a posttraumatic psychological intervention that emphasizes "talking through" as a means of processing psychological distress (B. Raphael, unpublished manuscript, 2001). Although there has been very strong belief in this process, there is little empirical evidence to suggest that debriefing as a form of intervention is helpful for general disaster-affected populations. Indeed, some research shows that it may add to the risk of adverse outcomes (e.g., Kenardy and Carr 2000; Kenardy et al. 1996).

Consensus conference members agreed that use of the single term *debriefing* to describe a broad range of mental health interventions (e.g., psychological debriefing, critical incident stress debriefing) is misleading. Conference members agreed that *debriefing* should be used only to describe operational debriefing (first developed by the military), which is a routine individual or group review of the details of an event from a factual perspective. Clearer descriptions of the interventions under investigation and more of an attempt to standardize interventions would aid in interpretation of research findings.

The studies reviewed in this section used interventions that the authors described as debriefing interventions. Most of these interventions are rooted in critical incident stress debriefing

(CISD) (Mitchell 1983), which was developed to provide education, ventilation, and support for emergency service personnel in group settings. CISD is a formalized, structured method of group review of the stressful experience of a disaster conducted in the first few days (up to 48–72 hours after the event). *Psychological debriefing* refers to less formalized processes of debriefing than does CISD. It includes education and review processes (Dunning 1988; Raphael 1977) and often includes a positive focus on resilience and coping strategies. There is no systematic research for psychological debriefing as an operationalized intervention, nor has psychological debriefing been clearly differentiated from CISD in research studies.

Mitchell and Everly (2000) recently reconceptualized debriefing as a broader crisis intervention technique for use beyond emergency services workers. They acknowledge that there is a need for greater methodological rigor in studies of debriefing, and they suggest that CISD has not been sufficiently evaluated in methodologically rigorous studies.

Debriefing Studies for General Population Samples

Evidence from RCTs to date has shown that CISD is associated with either a lack of significant benefits or more adverse outcomes for those debriefed. Rose et al. (2000), having reviewed the few well-controlled and well-designed trials on CISD, concluded that there is inadequate evidence to support the continuing use of debriefing. In another review of debriefing RCTs, Litz et al. (in press) recommended against the use of single-session debriefing and cited a need for more research on debriefing. Of six well-designed debriefing RCTs chosen for inclusion in our review, three (Conlon et al. 1999; Lee et al. 1996; Rose et al. 1999) found that individuals who were offered one-session debriefing interventions did not have better symptomatic outcomes than did a no-intervention control group. In the other three studies (Bisson et al. 1997; Hobbs et al. 1996; Mayou et al. 2000), participants in the one-session debriefing group actually fared worse than did participants in a no-intervention group. None of these six studies was conducted with disaster-affected populations. Given the weight of the evidence, one might conclude that debriefing should not be implemented within the first month after trauma. There are serious methodological problems, however, in all three RCTs that found debriefing to be associated with more severe symptoms. Most importantly, in all three studies, individuals in the debriefed groups had more severe injuries initially or longer hospital stays than did individuals in the nondebriefed groups (Bisson et al. 1997; Hobbs et al. 1996; Mayou et al. 2000).

Debriefing for Emergency Personnel and the Military

CISD has had its strongest proponents within the emergency responder and military communities. All studies discussed as follows have methodological limitations that are serious enough to warrant extreme caution in generalizing from the findings. Described are the most relevant debriefing studies with emergency and military personnel, with significant limitations noted.

Eight studies were identified that included a comparison of debriefed versus nondebriefed disaster- or war-exposed emergency or military personnel on posttraumatic sequelae (Carlier et al. 1998, 2000; Deahl et al. 1994, 2000; Eid et al. 2001; Hytten and Hasle 1989; Jenkins 1996; Kenardy et al. 1996). Most of these studies, being naturalistic, consequently have inevitable methodological limitations such as lack of treatment adherence measures or randomization. Self-selection for debriefing, which poses a significant threat to internal validity, was present in four of these studies (Carlier et al. 2000; Hytten and Hasle 1989; Jenkins 1996; Kenardy et al. 1996). Only one of the eight studies included an attempt at randomization, and the strategy used was somewhat problematic (Deahl et al. 2000). Four of the eight studies yielded no differences in symptoms between the debriefed and nondebriefed groups (Carlier et al. 2000; Deahl et al. 1994, 2000; Hytten and Hasle 1989), two showed worse symptoms in the debriefed group (Carlier et al. 1998; Kenardy et al. 1996), and two showed more favorable outcomes in the debriefed group (Eid et al. 2001; Jenkins 1996).

Conclusions About Debriefing as a Potential Early Intervention After Mass Violence

Despite widespread application of stress debriefing, there is little empirical evidence of its effectiveness for civilian populations affected by disasters (Raphael and Wilson 2000).

A consistent trend in all of the studies we reviewed is that debriefing has not been associated with better clinical outcomes. Available evidence shows that in some instances it may actually complicate recovery. If these negative findings are accepted, it is instructive to consider why debriefing may be ineffective or problematic. The following hypotheses have been put forth (Raphael 2001):

- Multiple and complex stressors with different time lines are not appropriately addressed by one-session debriefings.
- Heightened arousal generated by recitation of traumatic experiences during the debriefing process may cause physiological hyperreactivity and the encoding of traumatic memories, both hallmarks of ASD and PTSD.
- Debriefing may be inappropriate for acute bereavement (Raphael et al. 2001).
- Debriefing may also increase the potential for retraumatization by hearing the stories of others and may possibly interfere with habituation (Foa et al. 2000).
- There is a risk of stimulating excessive negative ruminations that may lead to depression (Solomon et al. 2000).
- There is a preference for individual, one-on-one (rather than group) interventions.
- The recommended 24- to 72-hour posttraumatic window for early debriefing intervention may be too short.
- Debriefing may be culturally inappropriate (Silove 2000; Weisaeth 2000).
- Debriefing may interfere with adaptation (e.g., avoidance) and natural recovery.
- The inadequate assessment of distress in the group setting may lead to the erroneous conclusion that such a one-time intervention has been sufficient to prevent further symptoms.

This may result in less monitoring and follow-up care than might have been the case if no debriefing had been implemented.

Practice guidelines on debriefing formulated by the International Society for Traumatic Stress Studies (Bisson et al. 2000) stipulate that there is little evidence that debriefing prevents psychopathology. The guidelines emphasize that debriefing is well received by participants and may be useful in terms of facilitating the screening of those at risk, disseminating education and referral information, and improving organizational morale. However, the guidelines also state that if it is employed, debriefing 1) should be conducted by experienced, well-trained practitioners, 2) should not be mandatory, 3) should use some clinical assessment of potential participants, and 4) should be accompanied by clear and objective evaluation procedures. The guidelines state that it is premature to conclude that debriefing should be discontinued, but "more complex interventions for those individuals at highest risk may be the best way to prevent the development of PTSD following trauma" (Bisson et al. 2000, p. 319).

There is clearly a need for much further systematic research in this field. Consensus conference participants concluded that "there is some Level 1 evidence suggesting that early interventions in the form of a single 1-to-1 recital of events and expression of emotions evoked by a traumatic event (as advocated in some forms of psychological debriefing) does not consistently reduce risks of later developing PTSD or related adjustment difficulties. Some survivors (e.g., those with high arousal) may be put at heightened risk for adverse outcomes" (National Institute of Mental Health 2002, p. 8).

Cognitive-Behavioral Interventions

At present, cognitive-behavioral interventions during the acute aftermath of trauma exposure appear to have the most promising results in preventing subsequent psychopathology. Four of five RCTs related to early cognitive-behavioral interventions (Bryant et al. 1998, 1999; Echeburua et al. 1996; Gidron et al. 2001) found clear superiority of the cognitive-behavioral therapy (CBT) group in reducing PTSD symptomatology compared with the experience of a control group, whereas one (Brom et al. 1993) did not. In addition, a controlled (but not randomized) comparison of CBT versus an assessment-only condition in the acute phase after trauma found fewer PTSD symptoms in the CBT group at a 5.5-month follow-up (Foa et al. 1995).

A study using a manualized, individual preventive intervention administered 1 month after a motor vehicle accident (MVA) (Brom et al. 1993) found no differences between those in the assessment-only control group and those in the intervention group on the Inventory of Events Scale. However, limitations of the study (e.g., variation in treatment length, more preintervention symptoms in the treatment group) make it difficult to draw firm conclusions about the efficacy of the intervention.

Foa and colleagues (1995) conducted a controlled (but not randomized) study testing brief CBT that was introduced in the acute aftermath of sexual and nonsexual assault. The matched control group received only assessment. Two months after assault, the CBT group endorsed fewer PTSD symptoms and only 10% of its members still met diagnostic criteria for PTSD, whereas 70% of the control group still had the disorder. At 5.5 months, there were few differences in PTSD symptom severity between groups, but the CBT group had significantly fewer reexperiencing of symptoms and depressive symptoms. The lack of significant differences in favor of the CBT group at 5.5 months appeared to be due to the small sample size and resultant lack of statistical power.

Echeburua et al. (1996) compared five 1-hour sessions of either combined (cognitive restructuring and specific coping skills) training or progressive relaxation training. Participants improved in both groups, with gains maintained at 12-month follow-up, although the combined treatment group showed less PTSD symptom severity than did control subjects at 12-month follow-up.

Bryant and colleagues (1998, 1999) conducted some of the best-controlled and most relevant studies of early intervention following potentially traumatizing events. They have shown that brief cognitive behavioral interventions introduced within the first month after a catastrophic event may not only ameliorate ASD but may also prevent the subsequent development of PTSD. Approximately 10 days after exposure to an MVA, an industrial accident, or a nonsexual assault, these researchers randomly assigned subjects with ASD to five individual 1.5-hour sessions of either a CBT or a supportive counseling control condition. In the earlier study (Bryant et al. 1998), the researchers found that fewer CBT subjects met criteria for PTSD after treatment and 6 months later. In the second study (Bryant et al. 1999), they compared two different individual CBT approaches (prolonged exposure plus anxiety management and prolonged exposure alone) to a supportive counseling intervention. They found that both CBT groups showed significantly greater reductions in PTSD symptom severity compared with those of the supportive counseling group.

Gidron et al. (2001) randomly assigned college students to either two sessions of an intervention rooted in CBT (memory structure intervention) via telephone or two sessions of a supportive listening (telephone) control condition within the first month after an MVA. Greater reductions in PTSD were observed in the CBT (memory structure intervention) group compared with those of the supportive listening group. Positive effects were still evident at a 3- to 4-month follow-up. Although the sample size was small and there was no long-term follow-up, this intervention certainly merits further study as a simple, cost-effective treatment for acutely traumatized individuals.

Possible Contraindications for Exposure Therapy

One powerful therapeutic component of the cognitive-behavioral techniques described is exposure therapy, in which the client is asked to retell the most stressful aspects of the traumatic event as if they are occurring at the present time. Bryant and Harvey (2000) suggest that exposure techniques may be contraindicated when the acutely traumatized client exhibits extreme anxiety, panic attacks, marked dissociation, borderline personality disorder, psychotic illness, anger as a primary trauma response, unresolved prior traumas, severe depression or suicide risk, complex comorbidity, substance abuse, marked ongoing stressors, or acute bereavement. When exposure therapy is contraindicated, other techniques such as anxiety management, cognitive restructuring therapy, or pharmacological intervention may be effective (Bryant and Harvey 2000). It should be noted that these contraindications are primarily theoretical and may change as the empirical literature on exposure therapies matures.

Eye Movement Desensitization and Reprocessing

No RCTs have been conducted to assess the effectiveness of eye movement desensitization and reprocessing (EMDR) within the first 4 weeks of traumatic exposure. Among adult survivors of Hurricane Andrew, EMDR that was introduced between 2.5 and 3.5 months after the disaster resulted in significant reductions in PTSD symptoms compared with the experience of a waiting-list control group (Grainger et al. 1997). Although the study has several methodological limitations, the use of an objective and reliable assessment battery as well as comparison with an untreated waiting-list control group makes these findings noteworthy.

Traumatic Grief

To date, there are no published studies on the treatment of traumatic grief or complicated bereavement specifically related to disaster situations. Until very recently, little distinction was drawn among complicated bereavement, traumatic grief, and normal grief reactions. As a result, research in the field lacks a unified definition of these terms, and inclusion criteria vary considerably from one study to another. The studies included in this review are RCTs that were conducted in the early phases after traumatic loss or that were based on inclusion criteria that addressed traumatic grief (Prigerson et al. 1999). The reader is referred to Jacobs and Prigerson (2000) for a more comprehensive review of the literature on traumatic grief.

In a pilot study of a CBT intervention tailored specifically for traumatic grief, Shear and colleagues (2001) found a large beneficial effect on grief, anxiety, and depressive symptoms. Although this was a pilot study with major limitations (e.g., no control group, high dropout rate), the large reduction in symptoms suggests that this approach warrants further study.

Raphael (1977) conducted an RCT within 2 months of onset of bereavement among widows who met high-risk criteria for postbereavement morbidity based primarily on poor social support networks, concurrent crises, and traumatic circumstances of death. The intervention group received a "nondirective, supportive" individual intervention with an average of four sessions. Significant differences were found between the groups, with more health impairment, doctor visits, weight loss, smoking, and alcohol intake in the control group.

Early Interventions for Children Exposed to Mass Violence or Disasters

As with adults, most of the empirically sound research that has been conducted with traumatized children has tested the efficacy of cognitive-behavioral interventions. It should be noted that most of the research in this area has been conducted with abused children with long-term symptoms (e.g., Berliner and Saunders 1996; Cohen and Mannarino 1996). Although the results of clinical trials of CBT with traumatized children are encouraging, the effect sizes are medium in size (Cohen et al. 2000). In the discussion that follows, we have included only the most relevant acute-phase treatments for children who have experienced disaster or other forms of single-incident traumas. In a few instances, we have included studies of later-stage interventions, due to their direct relevance to disaster situations. Much more research is needed in this area.

Yule and Udwin (1991) and Yule (1992) conducted a three-session (debriefing plus problem solving) intervention for 14- to 16-year-old children who had been involved in the sinking of a cruise ship. Ten days after the disaster, a debriefing session was conducted, followed by two problem-solving sessions targeting anxiety, avoidance, and intrusive thoughts. Data collected 5–9 months after the disaster indicated that students who received the intervention showed significantly lower fear and anxiety scores than did children from a comparison school who did not undergo debriefing. The major methodological limitation of this study was the lack of random assignment and the unclear nature of the treatment itself.

Field and colleagues (1996) evaluated the effectiveness of massage therapy for children exposed to Hurricane Andrew within 1 month of the disaster. Children were randomly assigned to either viewing a neutral videotape with a graduate student or receiving back massage therapy, each for 30 minutes twice a week for a month. Children in the massage therapy condition showed greater reductions in anxiety and depression and greater increases in relaxation. Although methodological limitations make interpretation of results difficult, it is intriguing that an intervention for children that promoted general relaxation and did not include any cognitive-behavioral components was helpful in reducing symptoms of general distress. Unfortunately, this study did not include a specific measure of PTSD and did not have adequate treatment adherence measures.

Although they were not conducted in the immediate aftermath of trauma, school-based CBT interventions such as those studied by Goenjian and colleagues (1997) after the Armenian earthquake and by March and colleagues (1998) after single-incident traumas (e.g., MVAs) warrant replication in acute trauma situations. Both of these studies yielded reductions in PTSD, depression, anxiety, and anger scores after treatment.

Pharmacotherapy

Although psychopharmacological research in the area of PTSD is growing, there are only a few well-designed studies that have examined the effects of medications in the very early phases after trauma. The most important and best-designed study on pharmacotherapy for acutely traumatized individuals was carried out by Robert and colleagues (1999), who used a prospective, randomized, double-blind design to test whether children with burn injuries and ASD symptoms might benefit from imipramine treatment administered for 7 days or more after they were injured. Imipramine was significantly more effective than chloral hydrate, with 83% of children who received low-dose imipramine treatment showing a reduction in ASD symptoms, in contrast to 38% of the chloral hydrate group.

Pitman and colleagues (2002) tested whether PTSD symptoms could be prevented among adult survivors of acute trauma who were given a 10-day, double-blind course of the β-adrenergic antagonist propranolol (40 mg 4 times/day) versus a 10-day course of placebo. Forty-one emergency room patients who had just experienced a traumatic event as defined in DSM-IV were recruited for the randomized, double-blind study. The treatment and control groups did not differ in terms of PTSD symptoms at either a 1-month or a 3-month assessment. Despite the fact that the groups did not differ in concentration of PTSD cases, 0% of the propranolol patients versus 43% of the placebo patients were classified as physiological responders 3 months after the event when tested in the laboratory with a script-driven imagery protocol based on the traumatic event to which they had been exposed. This pilot study has important theoretical implications and suggests that larger studies with a longer-term follow-up are warranted.

Gelpin and colleagues (1996) conducted a small pilot study in which the benzodiazepines clonazepam and alprazolam were prescribed approximately 7 days after patients visited an emergency room for treatment related to potentially traumatic life events. At the 6-month assessment, nine participants in the benzodiazepine group (69%), versus two in the control group (15%), met the diagnostic criteria for PTSD according to the Clinician-Administered PTSD Scale, suggesting that benzodiazepine treatment may have actually worsened outcomes. This result is consistent with other negative results involving benzodiazepine treatment for chronic PTSD (Friedman et al. 2000). To date, there is no evidence that benzodiazepines are an effective pharmacological intervention for people with either acute or chronic posttraumatic reactions.

Stanovic and colleagues (2001) reported that burn victims treated with a low dose of risperidone experienced diminished nightmares and flashbacks and decreased hyperarousal and sleep disturbances 1–2 days after starting treatment. Although this was a small retrospective pilot study, the results warrant the performance of a prospective study to better understand the efficacy of the use of risperidone in treating early traumatic stress symptoms.

Longer-term studies of pharmacotherapy for PTSD may have relevance for acute interventions. Almost every class of psychotropic agent has been prescribed for PTSD patients. The best evidence supports the use of selective serotonin reuptake inhibitors (SSRIs) as first-line medications for PTSD. Recent studies with sertraline (Davidson et al. 2001a, 2001b; Londborg et al. 2001; Rapaport et al. 2002) and paroxetine (Marshall et al. 2001; Tucker et al. 2001) indicate not only that these medications may reduce PTSD symptoms and produce global improvement in functioning but also that they are effective against comorbid disorders and associated symptoms and have few side effects. Other agents that have been used in chronic PTSD that might be effective for acutely traumatized individuals include non-SSRI antidepressants, antiadrenergic agents, anticonvulsants, and other atypical antipsychotic agents (Friedman et al. 2000).

In a recent review of pharmacological treatment of PTSD in children, Cohen (2001) notes that the use of psychopharmacological approaches is becoming more widespread despite a lack of double-blind, randomized, controlled trials. To date, there are no published reports of placebo-controlled medication trials that have been conducted in children diagnosed with PTSD. The best study regarding medications for traumatized children was the aforementioned RCT of imipramine for children with ASD symptoms. For a recent review of the open-label medication trials that have been conducted with children, the reader is referred to Cohen 2001 and Donnelly et al. 1999.

Conclusions

As can be seen in this review of the empirical literature, there are not enough well-controlled studies to strongly endorse any particular type of early intervention after mass casualties. Rather, consensus based on both empirical literature and experiential practice suggests the need for a multifaceted approach to the management of traumatic stress after disasters and mass violence. Such a strategy requires the coordination of interventions depending on a multitude of factors, including time elapsed since the incident and the level of impact of the event. At this time, for instance, there is strong initial evidence that for those most severely affected by a traumatic event, a brief 4- to 5-session cognitive-behavioral treatment introduced in the immediate aftermath may ameliorate ASD and prevent subsequent chronic psychopathology. However, use of this treatment in the early phases following disaster has not been systematically evaluated, and it may need to be modified for this context (R. Bryant, personal communication, 2002). On the other hand, RCTs on psychological debriefing currently suggest that this approach either is ineffective or may even exacerbate PTSD symptoms, but it has not been effectively evaluated for different audiences following disaster. Because there is essentially no research on either EMDR or pharmacotherapy as early interventions in the face of disasters, neither can be recommended at this time. There is certainly reason to hope that effective pharmacotherapeutic interventions for acute traumatic stress will be developed with time, given emerging findings on how traumatic stress affects brain function in both the short and the long term. The field of traumatic bereavement is in its infancy, and more research is needed before any conclusions can be drawn regarding specific interventions for traumatic grief.

Acute interventions with children have not been sufficiently tested empirically. However, research in this arena is developing rapidly, and it is to be expected that a stronger body of evidence related to early intervention with children will emerge within the foreseeable future. Based on the evidence showing the effectiveness of cognitive-behavioral interventions for children with chronic PTSD (Cohen et al. 2000), it is reasonable to expect that this approach will prove beneficial for acutely traumatized children as well.

As we consider the many specific components of early intervention, it is apparent that it is necessary to conduct dismantling studies that will rigorously evaluate the effectiveness of each separate component, especially with respect to the optimal timing of such interventions. The range of component practices requiring systematic evaluation includes practices such as debriefing, education, outreach, needs assessment, triage, and formal clinical interventions. It is necessary to determine whether current practices are effective in ameliorating specific outcomes, or whether new interventions should be designed to accomplish such objectives. Other challenges include the development and implementation of efficient and accurate procedures for identifying individuals who are at high risk for progressing to chronic posttraumatic problems (Brewin et al. in press).

There is also a need for research that addresses the potential breadth and complexity of early intervention by including individuals with comorbid conditions, by examining different survivor groups, and by sampling varied service delivery settings (e.g., shelters, first aid stations, clinics, and hospitals). There is a related need to examine a range of outcomes, including not only PTSD, but also problems such as substance abuse, depression, anger, violence, interpersonal functioning, and physical health. In addition to work that examines such individual outcomes, research is needed that focuses on group, organizational, and community outcomes. Examples of such outcomes include staff turnover, medical problems, organizational cohesion, morale, absenteeism, and performance deficits.

Future researchers will need to address the ethical issues involved in using traditional comparison groups such as no-treatment or waiting-list control groups after mass casualties. Providers have expressed concern that research assessment soon after mass traumatic events might exacerbate symptoms or be unacceptable to survivors (Ruzek and Zatzick 2000). Also, there is an understandable reluctance to assign survivors to comparison interventions that are believed to be less effective. Such reluctance clearly limits the conclusions that can be drawn from real-world disaster intervention studies. Within the field of traumatic stress, there has recently been a call to develop new research strategies that may be ethically acceptable without sacrificing scientific rigor. This appears to be an achievable goal (Ruzek and Zatzick 2000).

Although postdisaster mental health services have traditionally been delivered without systematic evaluation, it is hoped that an increased emphasis on early intervention research will result in the routine application of rigorous program evaluation to inform ongoing service improvement.

It is also important that the experiential knowledge of professional responders "in the trenches" continues to be synthesized and disseminated. Furthermore, the early intervention field needs to develop proactive, practical strategies for disseminating evidence-based information on intervention strategies to policy makers and practitioners in the field. Development and rigorous testing of effective early interventions and subsequent dissemination of such findings to frontline practitioners are critical goals at this time.

References

Berliner L, Saunders BE: Treating fear and anxiety in sexually abused children: results of a controlled 2-year follow-up study. Child Maltreat 1:294–309, 1996

Bisson JI, Jenkins PL, Alexander J, et al: Randomized controlled trial of psychological debriefing for victims of acute burn trauma. Br J Psychiatry 171:78–81, 1997

Bisson JI, McFarlane AC, Rose S: Psychological debriefing, in Effective Treatments for PTSD: Practice Guidelines From the International Society for Traumatic Stress Studies. Edited by Foa EB, Keane TM, Friedman MJ. New York, Guilford, 2000, pp 317–319

Brewin CR, Rose S, Andrews B: Screening to identify individuals at risk after exposure to trauma, in Early Intervention for Psychological Trauma. Edited by Schneider U. Oxford, Oxford University Press (in press)

Brom D, Kleber RJ, Hoffman MC: Victims of traffic accidents: incidence and prevention of post-traumatic stress disorder. J Clin Psychol 49: 131–140, 1993

Bryant RA, Harvey AG: Acute Stress Disorder: A Handbook of Theory, Assessment, and Treatment. Washington, DC, American Psychological Association, 2000

Bryant RA, Harvey AG, Dang ST, et al: Treatment of acute stress disorder: a comparison of cognitive-behavioral therapy and supportive counseling. J Consult Clin Psychol 66:862–866, 1998

Bryant RA, Sackville T, Dang ST, et al: Treating acute stress disorder: an evaluation of cognitive behavioral therapy and supportive counseling techniques. Am J Psychiatry 156:1780–1786, 1999

Carlier IVE, Lamberts RD, Van Uchelen AJ, et al: Disaster-related post-traumatic stress in police officers: a field study of the impact of debriefing. Stress Med 14:143–148, 1998

Carlier IVE, Voerman AE, Gerson BPR: The influence of occupational debriefing on post-traumatic stress symptomatology in traumatized police officers. Br J Med Psychol 73:87–98, 2000

Cohen JA: Pharmacologic treatment of traumatized children. Trauma, Violence, and Abuse 2:155–171, 2001

Cohen JA, Mannarino A: A treatment outcome study for sexually abused preschool children: initial findings. J Am Acad Child Adolesc Psychiatry 3:42–50, 1996

Cohen JA, Berliner L, March JS: Guidelines for treatment of PTSD: treatment of children and adolescents. J Trauma Stress 13:566–568, 2000

Conlon L, Fahy TJ, Conroy R: PTSD in ambulant RTA victims: a randomized controlled trial of debriefing. J Psychosom Res 46:37–44, 1999

Davidson J, Pearlstein T, Londborg P, et al: Efficacy of sertraline in preventing relapse of posttraumatic stress disorder: results of a 28-week double-blind, placebo-controlled study. Am J Psychiatry 158:1974–1981, 2001a

Davidson JR, Rothbaum BO, van der Kolk BA, et al: Multicenter, double-blind comparison of sertraline and placebo in the treatment of posttraumatic stress disorder. Arch Gen Psychiatry 58:485–492, 2001b

Deahl MP, Gillham AB, Thomas J, et al: Psychological sequelae following the Gulf War: factors associated with subsequent morbidity and the effectiveness of psychological debriefing. Br J Psychiatry 165:60–65, 1994

Deahl M, Srinivasan M, Jones N, et al: Preventing psychological trauma in soldiers: the role of operational stress training and psychological debriefing. Br J Med Psychol 73:77–85, 2000

Donnelly CL, Amaya-Jackson L, March JS: Psychopharmacology of pediatric posttraumatic stress disorder. J Child Adolesc Psychopharmacol 9:203–220, 1999

Dunning CM: Intervention strategies for emergency workers, in Mental Health Response to Mass Emergencies: Theory and Practice. Edited by Lystad M. New York, Brunner/Mazel, 1988, pp 284–307

Echeburua E, de Corral P, Sarasua B, et al: Treatment of acute posttraumatic stress disorder in rape victims: an experimental study. J Anxiety Disord 10:185–199, 1996

Eid J, Johnsen BH, Weisaeth L: The effects of group psychological debriefing on acute stress reactions following a traffic accident: a quasi-experimental approach. Int J Emerg Ment Health 3:145–154, 2001

Field T, Seligman S, Scafidi F, et al: Alleviating posttraumatic stress in children following Hurricane Andrew. J Appl Dev Psychol 17:37–50, 1996

Foa EB, Hearst-Ikeda DE, Perry KJ: Evaluation of a brief cognitive-behavioral program for the prevention of chronic PTSD in recent assault victims. J Consult Clin Psychol 63:948–955, 1995

Foa EB, Keane TM, Friedman MJ (eds): Effective Treatments for PTSD: Practice Guidelines From the International Society for Traumatic Stress Studies. New York, Guilford, 2000

Friedman MJ, Davidson JRT, Mellman TA, et al: Pharmacotherapy, in Effective Treatments for PTSD: Practice Guidelines From the International Society for Traumatic Stress Studies. Edited by Foa EB, Keane TM, Friedman MJ. New York, Guilford, 2000, pp 326–329

Gelpin E, Bonne OB, Peri T, et al: Treatment of recent trauma survivors with benzodiazepines. J Clin Psychiatry 57:390–394, 1996

Gidron Y, Gal R, Freedman SA, et al: Translating research findings to PTSD prevention: results of a randomized-controlled pilot study. J Trauma Stress 14:773–780, 2001

Goenjian AK, Karayan I, Pynoos RS, et al: Outcome of psychotherapy among early adolescents after trauma. Am J Psychiatry 154:536–542, 1997

Grainger RD, Levin C, Allen-Byrd L, et al: An empirical evaluation of eye movement desensitization and reprocessing (EMDR) with survivors of a natural disaster. J Trauma Stress 10:665–671, 1997

Hobbs M, Mayou R, Harrison B, et al: A randomized trial of psychological debriefing for victims of road traffic accidents. BMJ 313:1438–1439, 1996

Hytten K, Hasle A: Fire fighters: a study of stress and coping. Acta Psychiatr Scand Suppl 355:50–55, 1989

Jacobs SC, Prigerson H: Psychotherapy of traumatic grief: a review of evidence for psychotherapeutic treatments. Death Stud 24:479–495, 2000

Jenkins SR: Social support and debriefing efficacy among emergency medical workers after a mass shooting incident. J Soc Behav Pers 11:477–492, 1996

Kenardy JA, Carr VJ: Debriefing post disaster: follow-up after a major earthquake, in Psychological Debriefing: Theory, Practice and Evidence. Edited by Raphael B, Wilson JP. Cambridge, Cambridge University Press, 2000, pp 174–181

Kenardy JA, Webster RA, Lewin TJ, et al: Stress debriefing and patterns of recovery following a natural disaster. J Trauma Stress 9:37–49, 1996

Lee CW, Gavriel H, Richard J: Eye movement desensitization: past research, complexities, and future directions. Aust Psychol 31:168–173, 1996

Litz BT, Gray MJ, Bryant RA, et al: Early intervention for trauma: current status and future directions. Clinical Psychology: Science and Practice 9:112–134, 2002

Londborg PD, Hegel MT, Goldstein S, et al: Sertraline treatment of posttraumatic stress disorder: results of 24 weeks of open-label continuation treatment. J Clin Psychiatry 62:325–331, 2001

March JS, Amaya-Jackson L, Murray MC, et al: Cognitive-behavioral psychotherapy for children and adolescents with posttraumatic stress disorder after a single-incident stressor. J Am Acad Child Adolesc Psychiatry 37:585–593, 1998

Marshall RD, Beebe KL, Oldham M, et al: Efficacy and safety of paroxetine treatment for chronic PTSD: a fixed-dose, placebo-controlled study. Am J Psychiatry 158:1982–1988, 2001

Mayou R, Ehlers A, Hobbs M: Psychological debriefing for road traffic accident victims: three-year follow-up of a randomized controlled trial. Br J Psychiatry 176:589- 593, 2000

Mitchell JT: When disaster strikes: the critical incident stress debriefing process. J Emerg Med Serv 8:36–39, 1983

Mitchell JT, Everly GS: Critical incident stress management and critical incident stress debriefings: evolutions, effects and outcomes, in Psychological Debriefing: Theory, Practice and Evidence. Edited by Raphael B, Wilson J. Cambridge, Cambridge University Press, 2000, pp 71–90

National Institute of Mental Health: Mental Health and Mass Violence: Evidence-Based Early Psychological Intervention for Victims/Survivors of Mass Violence. A Workshop to Reach Consensus on Best Practices (NIH Publ No 02-5138). Washington, DC, U.S. Government Printing Office, 2002

Norris FH, Friedman MJ, Watson PJ, et al: 60,000 disaster victims speak, Part I. An empirical review of the empirical literature: 1981–2001. Psychiatry 65:207–239, 2002

North CS, Nixon SJ, Shariat S, et al: Psychiatric disorders among survivors of the Oklahoma City bombing. JAMA 282:755–762, 1999

Pitman RK, Sanders KM, Zusman RM, et al: Pilot study of secondary prevention of posttraumatic stress disorder with propranolol. Biol Psychiatry 51:189–192, 2002

Prigerson HG, Shear MK, Jacobs SC, et al: Consensus criteria for traumatic grief: a preliminary empirical test. Br J Psychiatry 174:67–73, 1999

Raphael B: Preventative intervention with the recently bereaved. Arch Gen Psychiatry 34:1450–1454, 1977

Raphael B, Wilson J: Psychological Debriefing: Theory, Practice and Evidence. Cambridge, Cambridge University Press, 2000

Raphael B, Minkov C, Dobson M: Psychotherapeutic and pharmacological intervention for bereaved persons, in Handbook of Bereavement Research: Consequences, Coping, and Care. Edited by Stroebe MS, Hansson RO, Stroebe W, et al. Washington, DC, American Psychological Association, 2001, pp 587–612

Rapaport MH, Endicott J, Clary CM: Posttraumatic stress disorder and quality of life: results across 64 weeks of sertraline treatment. J Clin Psychiatry 63:59–65, 2002

Robert R, Blakeney PE, Villarreal C, et al: Imipramine treatment in pediatric burn patients with symptoms of acute stress disorder: a pilot study. J Am Acad Child Adolesc Psychiatry 38:873–878, 1999

Rose S, Brewin CR, Andrews B, et al: A randomized controlled trial of individual psychological debriefing for victims of violent crime. Psychol Med 29:793–799, 1999

Rose S, Bisson JI, Wessely SC: Psychological debriefing for preventing post traumatic stress disorder (PTSD). Cochrane Database Syst Rev 4:CD000560, 2001

Ruzek JI, Zatzick DF: Ethical considerations in research participation among acutely injured trauma survivors: an empirical investigation. Gen Hosp Psychiatry 22:27–36, 2000

Shear MK, Frank E, Foa E, et al: Traumatic grief treatment: a pilot study. Am J Psychiatry 158:1506–1508, 2001

Silove D: A conceptual framework for mass trauma: implications for adaptation, intervention and debriefing, in Psychological Debriefing: Theory, Practice and Evidence. Edited by Raphael B, Wilson JP. Cambridge, Cambridge University Press, 2000, pp 337–350

Solomon Z, Neria Y, Witztum E: Debriefing with service personnel in war and peace roles: experience and outcomes, in Psychological Debriefing: Theory, Practice and Evidence. Edited by Raphael B, Wilson JP. Cambridge, Cambridge University Press, 2000, pp 161–173

Sprang G: Coping strategies and traumatic stress symptomatology following the Oklahoma City bombing. Social Work and Social Sciences Review 8:207–218, 2000

Stanovic JK, James KA, VanDevere CA: The effectiveness of risperidone on acute stress symptoms in adult burn patients: a preliminary retrospective pilot study. J Burn Care Rehabil 22:210–213, 2001

Tucker P, Zaninelli R, Yehuda R, et al: Paroxetine in the treatment of chronic posttraumatic stress disorder: results of a placebo-controlled, flexible-dosage trial. J Clin Psychiatry 62:860–868, 2001

Weisaeth L: Briefing and debriefing: group psychological interventions in acute stressor situations, in Psychological Debriefing: Theory, Practice and Evidence. Edited by Raphael B, Wilson, JP. Cambridge: Cambridge University Press, 2000, pp 43–57

Yule W: Post-traumatic stress disorder in child survivors of shipping disasters: the sinking of the 'Jupiter.' Psychother Psychosom 57:200–205, 1992

Yule W, Udwin O: Screening child survivors for post-traumatic stress disorders: experiences from the 'Jupiter' sinking. Br J Clin Psychol 30:131–138, 1991

Chapter 5

Terrorism With Weapons of Mass Destruction

Chemical, Biological, Nuclear, Radiological, and Explosive Agents

Robert J. Ursano, M.D.
Ann E. Norwood, M.D.
Carol S. Fullerton, Ph.D.
Harry C. Holloway, M.D.
Molly Hall, M.D.

The use of weapons of mass destruction by terrorists gained international attention after the Japanese cult Aum Shinrikyo released sarin gas in the Tokyo subway system in 1995. Concern was heightened when it was learned that the group had also (unsuccessfully) released anthrax and had attempted to obtain the Ebola virus. In the United States, the terrorist attacks of September 11th, 2001, and the letters containing anthrax spores that were mailed to media outlets and government officials in October that same year shattered Americans' belief that they were immune from such events. Although the terrorist attacks themselves were circumscribed, the psychological impact was widespread, resulting in a variety of psychological responses throughout the world. Because the ultimate goals of terrorism are psychological and behavioral, psychiatrists can make valuable contributions in helping their communities prepare for and respond to such attacks. In this chapter, we review individual and community psychological and behavioral responses to terrorist attacks using these novel weapons of mass destruction. At the time this chapter was written, terrorists had successfully used only sarin (Japan) and anthrax (United States), and little had been published in the scientific literature on the psychological consequences of the anthrax attacks. Therefore, selected material from analogous events such as natural outbreaks and accidents are also presented for illustrative purposes.

Terrorism

There is no single definition of terrorism recognized by government agencies. Terrorism refers to a threat or action that creates terror or horror and is undertaken to achieve a political, ideological, or theological goal. Terrorism represents a special type of a disaster—one caused by human malevolence, which produces higher rates of psychiatric casualties than do natural disasters or technological accidents (North 1995). Terrorists intend to disrupt society by creating intense fear and disorganization. They seek to violate basic expectations of everyday life by attacking sites of government, work, recreation, and worship. These acts shatter usual predictable routines, people's beliefs in a just world, and people's sense of personal and community safety.

The primary goal of terrorism is to create terror. This simple but often forgotten element means that the target of terrorism is not only those who are killed, injured, or even directly affected. The target is an entire nation—in the United States, nearly 300 million people. Therefore, there are three populations of concern for mental health professionals and psychiatrists in particular: 1) those directly exposed, who may become ill with posttraumatic stress disorder (PTSD), depression, and alcohol use; 2) those who were vulnerable before the event and now must manage their lives with fewer resources (for example, the loss of child care or a much longer commute)—such losses of social supports may tip the vulnerable over the edge of illness; and 3) the potentially millions who experience an altered sense of safety and hypervigilance. All three of these populations require help. The tools for reaching these different groups and their needs are different, but all require attention.

Weapons of Mass Destruction

Although there have been thousands of terrorist attacks throughout the world using conventional weapons, the use of weapons of mass destruction—in particular chemical and biological agents—is a relatively new phenomenon. The term *weapons of mass destruction* is problematic, however. Chemical, biological, and radiological agents can produce mass destruction, but in the future they likely will be used more commonly as weapons of mass disruption. These weapons can be used in a manner that produces relatively few fatalities but that produces substantial psychological, social, and economic harm (Hyams et al. 2002). The term *chemical, biological, radiological, nuclear, and high-yield explosive* (CBRNE) agents is now used by many to designate the agents of interest without conjecture about their impact.

CBRN agents (that is, CBRNE agents excluding explosives) possess a number of unique characteristics that make them especially effective at creating terror. Conventional weapons produce immediate and tangible health consequences. In the immediate aftermath of a CBRN attack, however, one often cannot determine whether or not one has been injured. Most CBRN agents are invisible and odorless. Many produce delayed illness and can be detected only by the use of special equipment.

These weapons have special psychological implications because they are imperceptible. The experience of feeling threatened or safe depends heavily on the information provided by the government and scientific experts. Most of this information is obtained through the mass media. Risk communication and news coverage revealing the relative efficacy of the efforts to manage consequences of an CBRN attack play a central role in how groups and individuals react: whether or not they perceive themselves at high or minimal risk, whether they have confidence in the government and medical response, and their determination of what protective actions should be taken.

The medical community and society in general have little experience with illnesses caused by these agents. This lack of familiarity heightens fear and apprehension, because it can be difficult to predict who will become ill and how the illness will evolve, especially when agents found in nature may have been modified.

These weapons are characterized by their potent traumatic stressors, which are associated with increased psychiatric morbidity. Some agents produce disfiguration, which amplifies fear and increases the psychological impact of the weapons. For example, the burns caused by vesicant agents such as mustard gas and the pustules resulting from smallpox are disquieting. Threat to life has been shown to be one of the most potent of psychological stressors, and all of these weapons have the potential to create morbidity and mortality on a grand scale. For many of these agents, the availability of medical treatment is limited, and in many cases, the effectiveness of treatment is uncertain because of the possibility that the agent has been modified. Biological agents that can be transmitted from person to person, such as plague and smallpox, can create widespread fear and anxiety because of rapid and broad dissemination in an age of global travel (Tables 5–1 and 5–2).

The weapons of terrorism also evolve. The novelty this produces can itself increase terror. Suicide bombings, shoes that explode, and trucks carrying high explosives create new hypervigilance. The use of jetliners as tools of terror was especially effective because it entailed the novel use of the familiar and the element of surprise.

Although high-yield explosives produce physical effects similar to those of conventional explosives, the psychological and social consequences are increased by an order of magnitude. The September 11 attacks on the World Trade Center, in particular, because of the scale of destruction and the large numbers of dead, had profound consequences, not just for those directly affected, but internationally.

Role of Psychiatrists

Events involving CBRNE agents represent special forms of disasters. Initially, all disasters are local events, because it takes time for state and federal agencies to respond and get in place. Therefore, it is important that psychiatrists have a grasp of the funda-

Table 5-1. Category A diseases

The U.S. public health system and primary health care providers must be prepared to address various biological agents, including pathogens that are rarely seen. High-priority agents include organisms that pose a risk to national security because they can be easily disseminated or transmitted from person to person; they result in high mortality rates and have the potential for major public health impact; they may cause public panic and social disruption; and they require special attention for public health preparedness.

Disease	Transmitted person to person	Infective dose (aerosol)	Incubation period	Duration of illness	Lethality (approx. case fatality rates)	Treatment/ vaccine efficacy (aerosol exposure)
Inhalation anthrax	No	8,000–50,000 spores	1–6 days	3–5 days (usually fatal if untreated)	High	Antimicrobial agents: ciprofloxacin or doxycycline Vaccine: 2 dose efficacy against up to 1,000 LD$_{50}$

Table 5–1. Category A diseases (*continued*)

Disease	Transmitted person to person	Infective dose (aerosol)	Incubation period	Duration of illness	Lethality (approx. case fatality rates)	Treatment/ vaccine efficacy (aerosol exposure)
Pneumonic plague	High	100–500 organisms	2–3 days	1–6 days (usually fatal)	High unless treated within 12–24 hours	Antibiotics: streptomycin, gentamicin, the tetracyclines, chloramphenicol Vaccine: 3 doses not protective against 118 LD_{50} in monkeys
Tularemia	No	10–50 organisms	2–10 days (average 3–5)	≥2 weeks	Moderate if untreated	Antibiotics Vaccine: 80% protection against 1–10 LD_{50}

Table 5–1. Category A diseases (continued)

Disease	Transmitted person to person	Infective dose (aerosol)	Incubation period	Duration of illness	Lethality (approx. case fatality rates)	Treatment/vaccine efficacy (aerosol exposure)
Smallpox	High	Assumed low (10–100 organisms)	7–17 days (average 12)	4 weeks	High to moderate	No proven treatment Vaccine: protects against large doses in primates
Viral hemorrhagic fevers	Moderate	1–10 organisms	4–21 days	Death between 7 and 16 days	High for Zaire strain, moderate with Sudan	No established treatment Vaccine: None
Botulism	No	0.001 μg/kg is LD_{50} for type A	1–5 days	Death in 24–72 hours; lasts months if not lethal	High without respiratory support	Antitoxin Vaccine: 3 dose efficacy 100% against 25–250 LD_{50} in primates

Source. Centers for Disease Control and Prevention 2002; U.S. Army Medical Research Institute of Infectious Diseases 2001.

Table 5–2. Category B diseases

Second-highest-priority agents include those that are moderately easy to disseminate; result in moderate morbidity rates and low mortality rates; and require specific enhancements of the Centers for Disease Control and Prevention's diagnostic capacity and enhanced disease surveillance.

Disease	Transmitted person to person	Infective dose (aerosol)	Incubation period	Duration of illness	Lethality (approx. case fatality rates)	Treatment
Brucellosis	No	10–100 organisms	5–60 days (usually 1–2 months)	Weeks to months	<5% untreated	Antibiotics: doxycycline, rifampin Vaccine: none
Cholera	Rare	10–500 organisms	4 hours–5 days (usually 2–3 days)	≥1 week	Low with treatment, high without	Fluid replacement Vaccine: no data on aerosol
Glanders	Low	Assumed low	10–14 days via aerosol	Death in 7–10 days in septicemic form	>50%	Limited information about antibiotic treatment Vaccine: none

Table 5–2. Category B diseases (*continued*)

Disease	Transmitted person to person	Infective dose (aerosol)	Incubation period	Duration of illness	Lethality (approx. case fatality rates)	Treatment
Q fever	Rare	1–10 organisms	10–40 days	2–14 days	Very low	Antibiotic: doxycycline Vaccine: 94% protection against 3,500 LD_{50} in guinea pigs
Venezuelan equine encephalitis	Low	10–100 organisms	2–6 days	Days to weeks	Low	No known treatment Vaccine: TC 83 protects against 30–500 LD_{50} in hamsters
Staphylococcal enterotoxin B	No	0.03 μg/person incapacitation	3–12 hours after inhalation	Hours	<1%	Vaccine: none

Table 5–2. Category B diseases *(continued)*

Disease	Transmitted person to person	Infective dose (aerosol)	Incubation period	Duration of illness	Lethality (approx. case fatality rates)	Treatment
Ricin	No	3–5 μg/kg is LD_{50} in mice	18–24 hours	Days; death within 10–12 days for ingestion	High	Vaccine: none
No category						
T-2 mycotoxins	No	Moderate	2–4 hours	Days to months	Moderate	No specific antidote, superactivated should be given orally if toxin is swallowed Vaccine: none

Source. Centers for Disease Control and Prevention 2002; U.S. Army Medical Research Institute of Infectious Diseases 2001.

mentals of disaster psychiatry to include the unique aspects of CBRNE agents.

Psychiatrists can play key roles in helping their communities prepare for terrorism and other disasters. They can help develop and review hospital disaster response plans, can serve as consultants to leaders to ensure that psychological and behavioral considerations are taken into account, and can help school systems in preparing to assist children and families in the event of an attack.

In the aftermath of an attack, psychiatrists may be asked to assist in performing triage on patients with mental status changes (DiGiovanni 1999). Consultation with health care providers, first responders, and others intensely exposed to traumatic stressors may be beneficial in sustaining the performance of these groups. Psychiatrists may also work with schools, civic organizations, public officials, and the media to educate and advise. Using a preventive medicine model of psychiatry, psychiatrists can help identify high-risk groups for surveillance and intervention (Pfefferbaum and Pfefferbaum 1998; Ursano et al. 1995). Although the area of acute intervention remains controversial, psychiatrists should familiarize themselves with the essential elements that characterize models commonly employed today as well as limitations and potential risks associated with their use. Patients with PTSD, depression, anxiety, and other psychiatric disorders often present to their primary care physicians with somatic complaints (Yehuda 2002). Psychiatrists should educate these colleagues on the recognition and treatment of these disorders as well as when to refer. Finally, psychiatrists can expect to treat the psychiatric sequelae of traumatic exposure over the longer term.

Institutions such as the U.S. Department of Defense and the Centers for Disease Control and Prevention have produced a wealth of excellent material on the diagnosis and treatment of disorders caused by CBRN agents; much of this information is available on the Internet. In Tables 5–1 through 5–3 we have distilled information on biological and chemical agents as a quick reference. Because there will continue to be further work in this area, psychiatrists need to stay abreast of advances in agent identification, protective measures, and treatment.

Table 5–3. Chemical warfare agents

U.S. Army code	Effects
Cyanides	
AC (hydrogen cyanide) CK (cyanogen chloride)	All cyanides produce progressive histotoxic tissue hypoxia. CK produces irritation of the eyes and mucous membranes. Exposure to high concentrations of gas results in initial hyperpnea, followed by loss of consciousness, apnea, cessation of cardiac activity, and death. Low concentrations of gas effects are slower.
Nerve agents	
GA (tabun) GB (sarin) GD (soman) GF VX	Small exposure produces miosis; rhinorrhea; slight bronchoconstriction; secretions (slight dyspnea) Moderate exposure produces miosis; rhinorrhea; bronchoconstriction; secretions (moderate to marked dyspnea) Large exposure is the same as moderate exposure, plus loss of consciousness, convulsions (seizures), generalized fasciculations, flaccid paralysis, and apnea; involuntary micturition and defecation are possible with seizures.
Lung toxicants	
CG (phosgene) DP (diphosgene)	Toxic inhalants may cause damage in one or more ways: asphyxiation; topical damage to the respiratory tract; cellular damage with consequent airway obstruction, pulmonary interstitial damage, or alveolar capillary damage; systemic damage with consequent damage to other organ systems; or allergic response resulting in pulmonary or systemic reaction.

Table 5–3. Chemical warfare agents *(continued)*

U.S. Army code	Effects
Lung toxicants *(continued)*	
	In the first 30 minutes after exposure, low concentrations may produce mild cough, a sense of chest discomfort, and dyspnea. Moderate concentrations cause lacrimation and the unique complaint that smoking tobacco produces objectionable taste. High concentrations may cause rapidly developing pulmonary edema with severe cough, dyspnea, and frothy sputum.
Vesicants	
HD (mustard)	Produces pain hours later, results in immediate tissue damage and onset of clinical effects hours later; produces fluid-filled blister.
L (lewisite)	Produces immediate pain; tissue damage in
HL	seconds to minutes; results in fluid-filled blister.
Incapacitating agent	
BZ	Most conspicuous signs are peripheral symptoms of tachycardia, dryness of skin and mucous membranes, and moderately elevated blood pressure. Incoordination, confusion, and slurred speech appear early. Mydriasis, stupor, and coma may develop. After many hours have elapsed, peripheral cholinergic blockade may have largely subsided. Bizarre behavior (e.g., groping, undressing, mumbling) and failure to follow commands or conversation may be the most conspicuous feature.

Table 5–3. Chemical warfare agents *(continued)*

U.S. Army code	Effects
Incapacitating agent *(continued)*	
	Low dose results in mild delirium, represented by a drowsy state, occasional lapses of attention, and slight difficulty following complex instructions. Moderate dose results in moderate delirium, generally manifested by somnolence or mild stupor, indistinct speech, poor coordination, and generalized slowing in thought processes with some confusion and perplexity. High dose results in full syndrome of delirium results.
Tear gases	
CN	All tear gases cause burning and irritation,
CS	conjunctival injection, tearing, blepharospasm, and photophobia; burning and erythema of the skin. Gagging, retching, and vomiting may result; results in sneezing, coughing, tightness in the chest, irritation, and secretions; rhinorrhea and burning pain in the nose; and burning of mucous membranes and salivation in the mouth.
Vomiting gas	
DM (adamsite)	Headache, mental depression, chills, nausea, abdominal cramps, vomiting, and diarrhea may result and last for several hours after exposure.

Source. Adapted from Sidell et al. 1997.

Psychiatric Morbidity in the Wake of Events Involving CBRNE Agents

Terrorist attacks using conventional weapons such as guns and bombs have well-known psychiatric sequelae. PTSD was seen in roughly half of the patients 6 months after the 1987 Enniskillen bombing in Northern Ireland (Curran et al. 1990). In a study of French survivors of terrorist attacks, 18% of survivors were diagnosed with PTSD and 13% with major depression (Abenhaim et al. 1992). In a study of direct survivors of the Oklahoma City bombing in the United States, 34% had PTSD and 22% had major depression; 55% had no diagnosis, and nearly 40% of those with PTSD and depression had no previous psychiatric illness. The incidence of new cases of illness in those with no previous diagnosis can be expected to be highest in those directly exposed (North et al. 1999).

It is expected that like other kinds of disasters, events involving CBRN agents will result in psychiatric morbidity for some. People who were directly exposed may experience psychological distress; in addition, because of the uncertainty regarding who has been exposed and who may be attacked next, many unexposed individuals may also experience such distress. For most, these acute psychological reactions will resolve over time. However, for some, the reactions will not resolve and instead develop into symptoms of psychiatric disorders. Acute stress disorder (ASD), PTSD, depression, phobias, alcohol and nicotine abuse, and complicated bereavement will likely be encountered.

For most individuals, posttraumatic psychiatric symptoms following CBRNE terrorism are transitory. These early symptoms usually respond to receiving education, obtaining enough rest, and maintaining biological rhythms (e.g., sleeping at the same time, eating at the same time). Media exposure can be both reassuring and threatening. Limiting such exposure can minimize the disturbing effects, especially in children (Pfefferbaum et al. 2001). Providing education to spouses and significant others of those distressed can help in treatment as well as in identifying the worsening or persistence of symptoms.

PTSD is not uncommon after terrorist events. ASD and early PTSD may be more like the common cold—experienced at some time in life by nearly all. If they persist, they can be debilitating and require psychotherapeutic and pharmacological intervention. However, PTSD is neither the only trauma-related disorder nor even perhaps the most common (Fullerton and Ursano 1997; Norris 2002; North et al. 1999; Ursano 2002). People exposed to terrorism are at increased risk for developing depression, generalized anxiety disorder, panic disorder, and increased substance use (Breslau et al. 1991; Kessler et al. 1995; North et al. 1999, 2002). After a terrorist event, the contribution of the psychological factors to medical illness can also be pervasive—from heart disease (Leor et al. 1996) to diabetes (Jacobson 1996). Important is that injured survivors often have psychological factors affecting their physical condition (Kulka et al. 1990; North et al. 1999; Shore et al. 1989; Smith et al. 1990; Zatzick et al. 2001).

Traumatic bereavement (Prigerson et al. 1999); unexplained somatic symptoms (Ford 1997; McCarroll et al. 2002); depression (Kessler et al. 1999); sleep disturbance; increased alcohol, caffeine, and cigarette use (Shalev et al. 1990); and family conflict and family violence are not uncommon after traumatic events. Anger, disbelief, sadness, anxiety, fear, and irritability are expected responses. In each, the role of exposure to the traumatic event may be easily overlooked by a primary-care physician. Anxiety and family conflict can accompany the fear and distress of new terrorist alerts, toxic contamination, and the economic impact of lost jobs and companies' closing or moving. Medical evaluation that includes inquiring about family conflict can provide reassurance, can begin a discussion for referral, and can be a primary preventive intervention for children whose first experience of a disaster or terrorist attack is mediated through their parents.

Behavioral Responses to CBRN Agents: Areas of Special Concern

Overwhelming Medical Facilities

Case Example 1

After Iraq's invasion of Kuwait in 1990, Israeli officials began to prepare the public for missile attacks. Gas masks and autoinjectors of antidotes against nerve gas were distributed to the entire population (Karsenty et al. 1991). Israelis were advised to select a room in their homes and seal all its openings except an entrance door (Karsenty et al. 1991). The population was instructed to enter the sealed room and put on their gas masks if an alarm was sounded. Residents had between 4 and 5 minutes of warning between the sounding of the missile alarm and any impact. Between January 18 and February 28, 1991, there were 23 missile attack alerts, of which 5 proved to be false alarms. A total of 39 Iraqi missiles landed in Israel. A total of 1,059 people presented to Israeli emergency rooms in response to the alarms (including false alarms). Of these, 234 individuals (22%) were direct casualties of the missile explosions (232 people injured and 2 killed by the missile explosions), and the remaining 78% were behavioral and psychiatric casualties. These indirect casualties were composed of 544 patients (51%) with acute anxiety; 230 patients (22%) who had autoinjected atropine without exposure to agent; 40 (4%) who were injured while running to the sealed rooms; and 11 who died (1%)—7 who suffocated due to leaving the filter closed on their gas masks and 4 who died of intercurrent myocardial infarctions (Karsenty et al. 1991). The number of patients presenting with anxiety or unneeded injections of atropine were highest after the initial missile attack alarms and decreased over time (Karsenty et al. 1991). Another finding was that psychological reactions were found to be almost twice as high when the patient was alone or with only one other person in the sealed room (Karsenty et al. 1991). The use of a bedroom as the sealed room was also associated with a lower frequency of psychological reactions (Karsenty et al. 1991). The Israeli experience with the threat of the use of chemical weapons is consonant with the Japanese findings of substantial symptoms of anxiety and autonomic arousal following actual exposure or belief of exposure to chemical weapons.

Case Example 2

The Aum Shinrikyo cult launched two successful attacks using sarin gas. In June 1994, sarin was used in Matsumoto, Japan, resulting in 7 deaths and more than 200 injuries. On March 20, 1995, five 2-person teams placed plastic pouches hidden in newspapers on three subway lines that were converging at major subway stations in Tokyo (Tucker 1996). The pouches contained liquid sarin, an organophosphate nerve agent, which evaporated slowly after the terrorists punctured the bags with sharpened umbrella tips (Tucker 1996). Passengers overcome by the fumes exited trains at 16 different stations along the three subway lines (Tucker 1996). The attack killed 11 people (passengers, firefighters, subway workers, and police officers) and resulted in more than 5,500 casualties (Bowler et al. 2001; Ohbu et al. 1997). In total, 1,046 people were admitted to 98 different hospitals because of visual symptoms, nausea, headache, cough, dyspnea, cardiac symptoms, and neuropathy (Bowler et al. 2001).

Events involving CBRN agents highlight the importance of the psychology of individual risk perception and how decisions to seek medical evaluation are made. Conventional terrorist weapons, such as explosives or guns, produce immediate and visible health consequences. Health care systems have a great deal of experience in managing these incidents on a small scale. There is little direct experience in the management of CBRN terrorism in the United States.

Based on the experiences in Israel and Japan, there is a concern that medical facilities may be initially overwhelmed by people seeking care, many of whom will not have actually been exposed. Belief that one has been exposed leads to the seeking of health care. One of the commonalities among events involving CBRN agents is the high proportion of people seeking medical assistance who are concerned that they have been exposed but for which no etiology for their symptoms is found. In Tokyo, for example, a very high proportion of the 5,000 patients who sought care were not admitted and had no signs of exposure (Ohbu et al. 1997). Many misattributed the signs and symptoms of anxiety and autonomic arousal to intoxication by sarin.

The rapid influx of noninjured as well as injured patients is a major concern, because the number of patients may overwhelm capacity. Triage to distinguish those who may be distressed from those who are injured is a critical first step in emergency care. Planners have struggled to devise a nonpejorative term to describe individuals who fear that they are ill but prove not to be. This group has been referred to using terms such as *psychological casualties, the worried well,* and other terms that are stigmatizing. The use of terms like these may result in inappropriate care, for example, determining through triage that individuals are psychological casualties before performing an adequate medical assessment.

Mass Sociogenic Illness

Case Example 3

In 1987 in Goiania, Brazil, two individuals who were scavenging for items to sell removed approximately 20 g (1,500 Ci) of cesium

137 from an old radiotherapy machine in an abandoned medical clinic. The machine was taken apart at the shop of a local junk dealer. The isotope attracted attention because it glowed in the dark, and it was given to friends and family members in the immediate vicinity (Collins and Bandeira de Carvalho 1993). A total of 249 people were contaminated internally or externally, and 4 died. All were relatives or neighbors of those who lived near the yard where the source had been disassembled or were employees or owners of the two junkyards to which pieces of the teletherapy unit had been taken (Brandao-Mello et al. 1991). Only those people in the four-block epicenter were exposed to radiation (Collins and Bandeira de Carvalho 1993), yet approximately 113,000 Goiania residents (10% of the city) sought screening. Of interest in planning triage, 11% of the 113,000 exhibited classic symptoms of radiation exposure (nausea, reddened skin, etc.) before being assessed (Collins 2002). After they were given a clean bill of health, their symptoms dissipated within a few hours (Collins 2002).

The occurrence of mass sociogenic illness in the wake of an attack with CBRN agents is a major concern for planners, who worry about the strain it will place on an already overburdened medical system. Mass sociogenic illness, also referred to as mass psychogenic illness and epidemic hysteria, is a social phenomenon in which two or more people share beliefs about a constellation of symptoms for which no identifiable etiology can be found (Boss 1997). This illness is typically triggered by an environmental event, often an odor or perceived odor, for which there is a robust emergency response. Individuals with unexplained symptoms attribute their illness to the environmental incident. These epidemics involve otherwise healthy people. In some instances, there may be group members with actual illness who are witnessed by individuals who then develop similar symptoms but without demonstrable pathology. Outbreaks of mass sociogenic illness have been reported after nuclear and chemical releases, incidents of excessive smog, and contamination of a water supply (Boss 1997). In the wake of September 11 and in a climate of fear of additional attacks, a series of outbreaks of mass sociogenic illness were reported. On September 29, 2001, paint fumes in a Washington state middle school triggered a bioterrorism scare in which 16 students and 1 teacher were medically evaluated (Wessely et al. 2001). On October 3, 2001, rumors of bioterrorism received on a short text service prompted more than 1,000 students in Manila, Philippines, to deluge clinics with complaints of flu-like symptoms (Wessely et al. 2001). Outbreaks of itchy red rashes that have occurred in more than two dozen elementary and middle schools across the United States since fall 2001 are also thought to represent mass sociogenic illness (Talbot 2002).

Panic

The word *panic* is often used to describe psychological responses to terrorism involving CBRNE agents. *Panic* refers primarily to a group phenomenon in which intense, contagious fear causes individuals to think only of themselves. They become paralyzed by fear or seek escape by any means necessary—"every man for himself." *Panic* also refers to an individual response that is characterized by the loss of rational thought due to overwhelming terror. A major goal of preparation for and response to events involving CBRNE agents is the prevention of panic and the preservation of individual, group, and community function.

Although panic does occur after disasters, it is rare. Surprise and novelty are risk factors for panic. Other factors include the belief that there is a small chance of escape; seeing oneself as being at high risk of becoming ill; limited resources that are available on a first-come, first-serve basis; a perceived lack of effective management of the catastrophe; and loss of credibility by authorities (Holloway et al. 1997).

The assumption that people will panic or become irrational after an attack with CBRNE agents has negative consequences. At times, authorities have provided inaccurate information and unfounded reassurances across a wide range of emergencies, including the recent anthrax attacks, motivated in part by a wish to calm the public. Ultimately, however, misleading statements and lying undermine credibility and contribute to even greater fear. The panic myth may also lead to neglect of the public's role in planning and responding to these events and missed opportunities to capitalize on the resourcefulness of nonprofessionals and civic organizations (Glass and Schoch-Spana 2002).

Responses of Hospital Staff and First Responders

In the United States, medical professionals have little experience in managing casualties resulting from releases of chemical, radiological, and biological agents. In the short term, physicians and other health professionals may experience fear, shock, anger, helplessness, and worries about their families and friends. Absenteeism is a major concern. In the 1994 outbreak of pneumonic plague in Surat, India, for example, 80% of the private physicians fled the city (Garrett 2000). An anonymous survey was conducted on the forty-first day of the Persian Gulf War in 42% of Israeli general hospitals. The questionnaire presented a scenario in which a spokesman for the Israel Defense Forces has announced that there has been a chemical warfare missile attack and has requested that hospital personnel report to duty. Questionnaires were distributed among all levels of hospital staff. Forty-two percent indicated that they would be willing to return to work (Shapira et al. 1991). For those unwilling to return to work, 75% cited concerns about personal safety as their primary reason (Shapira et al. 1991). Demoralization is also a concern if there are high mortality rates and an inability to provide adequate care for advanced illness. Familiarity with chemical and biological agents and training before the attack may enhance performance by the medical staff and help prevent breakdown. A realistic and well-rehearsed plan for dealing with events involving CBRNE agents will also help minimize feelings of helplessness and guilt about matters that could have gone more smoothly. Mental health consultation to hospital personnel can help ameliorate short-term distress and sustain functioning. Noncompliance with guidelines for use of personal protective equipment can create a significant health problem after CBRNE attacks (Fullerton and Ursano 1990).

Risk Communication

Multiple studies confirm that people assess risk and threat based on their feelings of control and their level of knowledge and familiarity with an event (for example, see MacGregor and Fleming 1996). Therefore, peanut butter is not sufficiently recognized as a risk to health and air travel is seen as overly risky (Slovic 1987). Widespread fear, uncertainty, and stigmatization are common after terrorist attacks and disasters. These fears require education about the actual risk and instruction in how to decrease risk, whether the risk is falling buildings in an earthquake or infection from a biological weapon. Instruction in active coping techniques can increase feelings of control and efficacy. In particular, fears of biological contagion or exposure to other contaminants can decrease community cohesion and can turn neighbor against neighbor as one tries to feel safe by identifying those who are exposed or ill as "not me."

As mentioned, the fear of exposure to toxic agents—including biological, chemical, and radiologic agents—can lead hundreds or even thousands to seek care, overwhelming hospitals and the health care system. Belief that one has been exposed to chemical and biological weapons leads individuals to seek health care and to change life patterns regardless of actual exposure.

Clear, accurate, and consistent information exchange is needed between health care professionals, government and local leaders, and the general public in times of a disaster. For medical and public health care professionals, explaining and describing risk is probably the most challenging situation for communicating with nonscientists. Key challenges include difficulties in translating scientific information, conflicts in risks and messages, and disagreements on the extent of the risk and how it should be assessed. Physicians have the ears of their community in their medical offices, at schools and community functions, and through the media; therefore, they are an important natural network for educating about risk and prevention.

Medical and behavioral health personnel should participate in the development of public information plans. Information from official and unofficial sources before, during, and after a disaster will shape expectations, behaviors, and emotional responses (Holloway et al. 1997). The delivery of consistent, updated information across multiple channels by way of widely recognized and trusted sources diminishes the extent to which misinformation can shape public attribution (Peters et al. 1997).

Special Issues Associated With Bioterrorism

Health care providers and the health care system are first responders in bioterrorism events. Bioterrorism differs from natural disasters in a number of fundamental ways. The microbial world is invisible and mysterious, and it can be frightening and unknown to many, including leaders, members of the media, and the general public. Bioterrorism is an act of human malice intended to injure and kill civilians and is associated with a higher rate of psychiatric morbidity than are so-called acts of God. A hurricane is usually an isolated event with subsequent consequences. Bioterrorism—due to the incubation period of microorganisms, and evolving echoes of exposure, fear, and possible spread of contagion—is a process trauma with consequences spread widely over time. In addition, there is the threat of further attacks, announced or covert. Bioterrorism is unbounded by time and space. Global travel can spread infected, asymptomatic individuals widely and quickly. The agents responsible for infectious diseases cannot be discerned by the unaided senses, which creates uncertainty and a sense of vulnerability and fear.

Bioterrorism can produce unfamiliar diseases that present challenges in diagnosis and treatment. The modern medical community has limited experience with the diseases produced by bioterrorism agents such as anthrax and smallpox virus. Naturally occurring outbreaks of infection may be difficult to distinguish from intentional attacks. Patient presentations and the at-risk populations differ in a terrorist attack from naturally occurring outbreaks because of the different routes of dissemination and possibly altered microorganisms.

Quarantine, forced evacuation, mandatory vaccination, and mandated treatment would curtail many civil liberties. The tendency to use these draconian measures increases as fear and anxiety increase. The demand for these actions as well as the failure to use them may contribute to community conflict and erode the public's confidence in the government. Careful analysis of the costs (including social costs) and benefits of these measures is needed.

Fear of contagion can have devastating consequences for all aspects of daily life after a bioterrorism event. The result may be that some communities become isolated and unable to obtain food and supplies. The lack of personnel due to infection or fear of infection can cripple basic community functions and financial institutions.

Important is that the economic and mental health impacts of bioterrorism occur in different sequences and phases than they do in natural disasters. Fear of contamination (warranted or unwarranted) creates second- and third-order effects such as the collapse of tourism and the flight of businesses soon after an event. Terrorist attacks will specifically target basic societal infrastructure such as transportation, mail delivery, and communication.

For all of these reasons, the mental health and behavioral effects of bioterrorism present substantial challenges for the health care system. The public health and mental health infrastructures have eroded to the point that they can barely meet requirements under normal circumstances. Many hospitals run short of beds during an average flu season. Ambulances are frequently diverted from urban emergency departments that have reached capacity. Changes in health care delivery have resulted in fewer hospital beds and just-in-time inventories, which have severely limited surge capacity for mass casualty events. Clinical care has been degraded because of the focus on episodic care rather than infrastructure development. The nationwide nursing shortage also hampers effective responses. The limited availability of treatment resources such as vaccines and antibiotics is also an impediment to a successful medical response to bioterrorism and to decreasing fear and anxiety. Normal care for hospital patients will necessarily be critically modified in a major bioterrorism attack, and elective treatments will be suspended entirely. Emergency care will be provided using a triage model that maximizes the efficient provision of care and bed utilization.

If contagious agents are used, many hospitals may have to close their doors to noninfected patients needing emergent care. Absenteeism can result from the conflicted loyalties of the hospital staff, divided between caring for their own families and taking care of patients. Developing plans to ensure that employees' families are cared for in the wake of a bioterrorism attack may diminish this absenteeism. Hospital bioterrorism response plans require provisions for supporting staff and for managing both expected and unexpected volunteers. Hospital staffs, police, and security personnel must be prepared to manage secure access to the hospital.

Sophisticated terrorists will understand that the agents that cause diseases in livestock and agriculture constitute important weapons that can produce devastating economic and psychological consequences. As seen in the United Kingdom, foot-and-mouth disease can rapidly spread to livestock in a wide geographic region, resulting in millions of dollars of losses. Bioterrorism attacks on livestock and agriculture will disproportionately affect the mental health of rural populations. Recent experiences with depopulation and carcass disposal after the outbreak of foot-and-mouth disease in the United Kingdom underscore the importance of integrating mental health into veterinary response. Agricultural preparedness and response should specifically incorporate psychological and behavioral expertise. For example, an important mental health preventive intervention can be working with veterinarians to encourage farmers and ranchers to freeze genetic materials so that important strains of plants and animals can be rebuilt after bioterrorism or a natural outbreak of disease. Mental health outreach to farmers and ranchers can be critical in coping with the losses caused by a bioterrorism attack.

It is important to remember that mental health intervention is a prompt and effective medical response to a bioterrorism attack. Early detection, successful management of casualties, and effective treatments bolster the public's sense of safety and increase confidence in institutions. Because the overriding goal of terrorism is to change people's beliefs, sense of safety, and behaviors, mental health experts are an essential part of planning and responding.

After a bioterrorism attack, the mental health needs of three populations must be addressed: those who are exposed and develop traditional psychiatric disorders, those with preexisting mental illness that may be reactivated or exacerbated, and the general population. The traditional airplane crash and natural disaster models of providing mental health services have limited applicability in bioterrorism. New models of monitoring shifting community mental health needs in real time, as well as innovative models for delivering care, are required. In these extreme environments, the use of telephone conferences, video teleconferences, and other technologies for providing mental health intervention can conserve limited resources and diminish disease transmission. Experts should help determine the skills needed for effective mental health preventive strategies and interventions. These skills can then be taught and refreshed across the medical training and education levels.

Communication, a core principle of mental health and behavioral care, is central to consequence management after a bioterrorism attack. The initial detection of disease begins a period of uncertainty in which the source of exposure, the scope of the outbreak, the number of people exposed, and the possibility of other agents being used are not fully known. The public's primary concern is about safety. Because biological agents are imperceptible, the public actively seeks information to gauge whether they are at risk and what steps they can take to protect themselves. There is a pressing need to hold repeated retreats with journalists, risk communication experts, and infectious disease specialists to craft consistent and practical educational messages for the public. These retreats can facilitate candid exchanges and establish ongoing relationships critical to responding effectively to a bioterrorism attack. These meetings can develop a common strategy for controlling the spread of false rumors, scapegoating, and conspiratorial theories.

Conclusions

The goal of terrorism is to disrupt the continuity of the nation by instilling fear and decreasing safety. This affects not only those who may develop mental health problems but also those who continue to work and care for their families and loved ones while experiencing an altered sense of safety, increased fear and arousal, and concern for their future. A number of factors influence group performance. Distrust before the event, a breakdown in communication, and the failure of critical elements can contribute to group disorganization. Poor leadership and a perception that there is no effective response can also contribute to mission failure. Consequence management for mental health begins with considering these needs of the nation, state, or locality as a whole and then moves to those directly exposed and those who may have been vulnerable before a terrorist attack and who now bear the additional burdens of lost supports and increased demands. Bioterrorism raises new and different behavioral and mental health issues. As part of the public health system, the mental health system must address needs for surge capacity and health surveillance so that it can best provide care for communities exposed to terrorism involving CBRNE agents, and in particular bioterrorism.

References

Abenhaim L, Dab W, Salmi LR: Study of civilian victims of terrorist attacks (France 1982–1987). J Clin Epidemiol 45:103–109, 1992

Boss LP: Epidemic hysteria: a review of the published literature. Epidemiol Rev 19:233–243, 1997

Bowler RM, Murai K, True RH: Update and long-term sequelae of the sarin attack in the Tokyo, Japan, subway. Chemical Health and Safety, January/February:1–3, 2001

Brandao-Mello CE, Oliveria AR, Valverde NJ, et al: Clinical and hematological aspects of 137Cs: the Goiania radiation accident. Health Phys 60:31–39, 1991

Breslau N, Davis GC, Andreski P, et al: Traumatic events and posttraumatic stress disorder in an urban population of young adults. Arch Gen Psychiatry 48:216–222, 1991

Centers for Disease Control and Prevention: Biological Diseases/Agents Listing. Atlanta, GA, Centers for Disease Control and Prevention, 2002. Available at http://www.bt.cdc.gov/Agent/Agentlist.asp. Accessed December 2, 2002

Collins DL: Human responses to the threat of or exposure to ionizing radiation at Three Mile Island, Pennsylvania, and Goiania, Brazil. Mil Med 167 (suppl 2):137–138, 2002

Collins DL, Bandeira de Carvalho A: Chronic stress from the Goiania 137Cs radiation accident. Behav Med 18:149–157, 1993

Curran PS, Bell P, Murray A, et al: Psychological consequences of the Enniskillen bombing. Br J Psychiatry 156:479–482, 1990

DiGiovanni CJ: Domestic terrorism with chemical or biological agents: psychiatric aspects. Am J Psychiatry 156:1500–1505, 1999

Ford CV: Somatic symptoms, somatization, and traumatic stress: an overview. Nord J Psychiatry 51:5–13, 1997

Fullerton CS, Ursano RJ: Behavioral and psychological responses to toxic exposure. Mil Med 155:54–59, 1990

Fullerton CS, Ursano RJ (eds): Posttraumatic Stress Disorder: Acute and Long-Term Responses to Trauma and Disaster. Washington, DC, American Psychiatric Press, 1997

Garrett L: Betrayal of Trust: The Collapse of Global Public Health. New York, Hyperion, 2000

Glass TA, Schoch-Spana M: Bioterrorism and the people: how to vaccinate a city against panic. Clin Infect Dis 34:217–223, 2002

Holloway HC, Norwood AE, Fullerton CS, et al: The threat of biological weapons: prophylaxis and mitigation of psychological and social consequences. JAMA 278:425–427, 1997

Hyams KC, Murphy FM, Wessely S: Responding to chemical, biological, or nuclear terrorism: the indirect and long-term health effects may present the greatest challenge. J Health Polit Policy Law 27:273–291, 2002

Jacobson AM: The psychological care of patients with insulin-dependent diabetes mellitus. N Engl J Med 334:1249–1253, 1996

Karsenty E, Shemer J, Alshech I, et al: Medical aspects of the Iraqi missile attacks on Israel. Isr J Med Sci 27:603–607, 1991

Kessler RC, Sonnega A, Bromet E, et al: Posttraumatic stress disorder in the National Comorbidity Survey. Arch Gen Psychiatry 52:1048–1060, 1995

Kessler RC, Barber C, Birnbaum HG, et al: Depression in the work place: effects of short-term disability. Health Aff (Millwood) 18:163–171, 1999

Kulka RA, Schlenger WE, Fairbank JA, et al: Trauma and the Vietnam War Generation: Report of Findings From the National Vietnam Veterans Readjustment Study. New York, Brunner/Mazel, 1990

Leor J, Poole WK, Kloner RA: Sudden cardiac death triggered by an earthquake. N Engl J Med 334:413–419, 1996

MacGregor DG, Fleming R: Risk perception and symptom reporting. Risk Anal 16:773–783, 1996

McCarroll JE, Ursano RJ, Fullerton CS, et al: Somatic symptoms in Gulf War mortuary workers. Psychosom Med 64:29–33, 2002

Norris FH: 60,000 disaster victims speak, Part I: an empirical review of the empirical literature, 1981–2001. Psychiatry 65:207–239, 2002

North CS: Human response to violent trauma. Baillière's Clinical Psychiatry 1:225–245, 1995

North CS, Nixon SJ, Shariat S, et al: Psychiatric disorders among survivors of the Oklahoma City bombing. J Am Med Sci 282:755–762, 1999

North CS, Tivis L, McMillen JC, et al: Psychiatric disorders in rescue workers after the Oklahoma City bombing. Am J Psychiatry 159:857–859, 2002

Ohbu S, Yamashina A, Takasu N, et al: Sarin poisoning on Tokyo subway. South Med J 90:587–593, 1997

Peters RG, Covello VT, McCallum DB: The determinants of trust and credibility in environmental risk communication: an empirical study. Risk Anal 17:43–54, 1997

Pfefferbaum B, Pfefferbaum RL: Contagion in stress: an infectious disease model for posttraumatic stress in children. Child Adolesc Psychiatr Clin N Am 7:183–194, 1998

Pfefferbaum B, Nixon SJ, Tivis RD, et al: Television exposure in children after a terrorist incident. Psychiatry 64:202–211, 2001

Prigerson HG, Shear MK, Jacobs SC, et al: Consensus criteria for traumatic grief: a preliminary empirical test. Br J Psychiatry 174:67–73, 1999

Shalev AY, Bleich A, Ursano RJ: Posttraumatic stress disorder: somatic comorbidity and effort tolerance. Psychosomatics 31:197–203, 1990

Shapira Y, Marganitt B, Roziner I, et al: Willingness of staff to report to their hospital duties following an unconventional missile attack: a state-wide survey. Isr J Med Sci 27:704–711, 1991

Shore JH, Vollmer WM, Tatum EL: Community patterns of posttraumatic stress disorders. J Nerv Ment Dis 177:681–685, 1989

Sidell FR, Takafuji ET, Franz DR: Medical aspects of Chemical and biological warfare, in Textbook of Military Medicine (series). Washington, DC, Office of the Surgeon General at TMM Publications, Borden Institute, Walter Reed Army Medical Center, 1997

Slovic P: Perception of risk. Science 236:280–285, 1987

Smith EM, North CS, McCool RE, et al: Acute postdisaster psychiatric disorders: identification of persons at risk. Am J Psychiatry 147:202–206, 1990

Talbot M: Hysteria hysteria. New York Times, June 2, 2002, p 42

Tucker JB: Chemical/biological terrorism: coping with a new threat. Politics Life Sciences 15:167–183, 1996

Ursano RJ: Post-traumatic stress disorder (editorial). N Engl J Med 346:130–131, 2002

Ursano RJ, Fullerton CS, Norwood AE: Psychiatric dimensions of disaster: patient care, community consultation, and preventive medicine. Harv Rev Psychiatry 3:196–209, 1995

U.S. Army Medical Research Institute of Infectious Diseases: Appendix C: BW agent characteristics, in Medical Management of Biological Casualties Handbook, 4th Edition, 2001, pp C-1–C-2

Wessely S, Hyams KC, Bartholomew R: Psychological implications of chemical and biological weapons. Br Med J 323:878–879, 2001

Yehuda R: Post-traumatic stress disorder. N Engl J Med 346:108–114, 2002

Zatzick DF, Kang SM, Hinton L, et al: Posttraumatic concerns: a patient-centered approach to outcome assessment after traumatic physical injury. Med Care 39:327–339, 2001

Index

*Page numbers printed in **boldface** type refer to tables or figures.*

Dioxin contamination, 44
Diphosgene, and chemical warfare, **136**
Disaster. *See also* Disaster responses; Trauma
children and sequelae of, 68–72, 113–114
definition of, 65–67
emotional development of children and, 72–77
empirical literature on effects of, 98–102
impact of on families, schools, and communities, 78–80
typology of, 37–38
Disaster responses, and psychiatric epidemiology. *See also* Disaster
bioterrorism and, 52–53
of children compared to adults, 63–65
course of mental health care and, 51–52
disaster response theory and, 37–42
guidelines for interventions and, 53–55
postdisaster populations and, 49–51
types of mental health care and, 42–49
Dissociation
diagnosis of ASD and, 3
neuropeptide Y and, 26
Distress. *See* Subdiagnostic distress
Dopaminergic system, and neurochemistry of PTSD and stress, 24
DSM-IV
acute stress disorder and, 2
definition of chronic PTSD in, 52

functional and organic mental disorders in, 30
DSM-IV-TR
definition of traumatic event, 1
diagnostic criteria for PTSD in, 43, 45, 50–51, 67
planning of mental health care and criteria for trauma-related diagnoses, 87
PTSD symptoms in, 4

Early interventions. *See also* Interventions
for children exposed to mass violence or disasters, 113–114
cognitive-behavioral therapy and, 109–112
effectiveness of, 117
eye movement desensitization and reprocessing, 112
general recommendations for, 104–105
key components of, 102–104
pharmacotherapy and, 114–116
psychological debriefing and, 105–109
research on, 97–98, 118–119
traumatic grief and, 112–113
Earthquakes, 47, 67. *See also* Armenian earthquake
Ebola virus, and bioterrorism, 125
Emergency personnel, and debriefing, 107. *See also* Firefighters; Rescue workers
Emotional development, of children, 72–77
Emotional memory, and neurobiology, 22–23

Lorazepam, and cholecystokinin (CCK), 27
Lung toxicants, and chemical warfare, **136–137**

Major depression. *See also* Depression
bioterrorism and, 139
in children after September 11, 2001, 83
comorbidity with PTSD in postdisaster settings, 46
Massage therapy, for children, 114
Mass destruction, weapons of, 127–128
Mass sociogenic illness, 142–144
Mass violence. *See also* Murder, mass
debriefing as early intervention after, 108–109
early interventions for children exposed to, 113–114
as type of disaster, 98
Mass Violence and Early Intervention conference (National Institute of Mental Health, 2002), 102, 104–105
Media
exposure of children to disasters and, 67, 90
psychiatric morbidity after bioterrorist events and, 139
Medical facilities. *See also* Health care system; Physicians
bioterrorism and overwhelming of, 140–142
responses of staff and professionals to terrorism, 145, 146

Medical illness, and psychological factors, 140
Medication. *See* Psychopharmacology
Memory
neurobiology of emotional, 22–23
reexperiencing as core symptom of PTSD and, 6–7
Mental health care. *See also* Interventions; Psychiatrists
bioterrorism and, 149–150
for children after September 11, 2001, 84–87
guidelines for postdisaster interventions and, 53–55
lessons learned from September 11, 2001 on planning of for children, 87–90
postdisaster response and course of, 51–52
postdisaster response and types of, 42–49
Meta-chlorophenylpiperazine (*m*-CPP), and serotoninergic system, 25–26
Military, and debriefing, 107. *See also* Combat-related PTSD; Veterans; War
Mineralocorticoid receptors, and neurochemistry of PTSD, 16, 19–20
Minnesota Multiphasic Personality Inventory, 48
Monitoring, and early interventions, 103
Moods, and signs of psychopathology after exposure to trauma, 2

War, impact of on children, 66. *See also* Combat-related PTSD; Military; Veterans

Weapons of mass destruction, 127–128

Weather-related disasters, 66. *See also* Cyclone Tracey; Hurricane Andrew

World Trade Center. *See* September 11, 2001

Worried well, and terrorism, 142

Yohimbine, and combat-related PTSD, 21